Masculinity, Meditation and Mental Health

Masculinity, Meditation and Mental Health

Tim Lomas

University of East London, UK

palgrave
macmillan

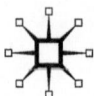

No portion of this publication may be reproduced, copied or transmitted
save with written permission or in accordance with the provisions of the
Copyright, Designs and Patents Act 1988, or under the terms of any licence
permitting limited copying issued by the Copyright Licensing Agency,
Saffron House, 6–10 Kirby Street, London EC1N 8TS.

Any person who does any unauthorized act in relation to this publication
may be liable to criminal prosecution and civil claims for damages.

The author has asserted his right to be identified as the author of this work
in accordance with the Copyright, Designs and Patents Act 1988.

First published 2014 by
PALGRAVE MACMILLAN

Palgrave Macmillan in the UK is an imprint of Macmillan Publishers Limited,
registered in England, company number 785998, of Houndmills, Basingstoke,
Hampshire RG21 6XS.

Palgrave Macmillan in the US is a division of St Martin's Press LLC,
175 Fifth Avenue, New York, NY 10010.

Palgrave Macmillan is the global academic imprint of the above companies
and has companies and representatives throughout the world.

Palgrave® and Macmillan® are registered trademarks in the United States,
the United Kingdom, Europe and other countries.

ISBN 978–1–137–34527–1

This book is printed on paper suitable for recycling and made from fully
managed and sustained forest sources. Logging, pulping and manufacturing
processes are expected to conform to the environmental regulations of the
country of origin.

A catalogue record for this book is available from the British Library.

A catalog record for this book is available from the Library of Congress.

For Kate,
and for my mother, father,
brother and sister

Contents

Acknowledgements

I feel truly grateful to have had the support and encouragement of some wonderful people without whom this book would not have been possible. First, I must thank my supervisory team at the University of Westminster, Damien Ridge, Tina Cartwright and Trudi Edginton. I could not have asked for more dedicated, caring, patient and thoughtful supervisors to guide me through this journey. I thank you for having faith in me, for reading through countless drafts with a critical yet always kindly eye, and for making me into a better student. Although I have written this book, in every sense it would not have been possible without you, and I consider this to be the product of all of our hard work over the last few years! I would also like to thank my colleagues at the University of East London, particularly Kate Hefferon and Itai Ivtzan, who have been so encouraging and supportive of me as I have embarked on my academic career, and who have helped me to develop my ideas. I am also very grateful to Nicola Jones at Palgrave Macmillan, who has been hugely important, having guided this book from inception to publication with great skill and enthusiasm.

A special word of thanks needs to go to the people who took part in the research that forms the substance of the book. I was overwhelmed by your open-hearted generosity in sharing your life stories with me. It was an honour to have met you all, and very inspiring. I hope you feel I have done justice to your amazing lives and characters. I am also very grateful to the Buddhist Centre for being so supportive of this research project, and for welcoming me into your community. Finally, words cannot do justice to the gratitude I feel to the people who are very closest to me, whose love and support is the very basis for my life, let alone this book. To mum and dad, just thank you for everything. You are my foundation and my inspiration, and I owe you everything. To Peter and Lauren, thank you for being the best brother and sister, for all the love and support, for all the good times, and just for being there for me. And, to Kate, love of my life, best friend and soul mate. You are my sunshine, and have made me happier than I thought it possible to be. Thank you for all the encouragement and support, the patience with my long hours, and the love and care (and delicious food!) that has given me nourishment and sustenance in every way. I could not have done this without you. You are all the best family one could wish for, and I love you more than I can possibly express.

Introduction

[As a youth] I was trying to emulate some kind of manhood, seeking symbols of machoism, sexual conquests, being anarchic, not conforming. A lot of that came from feeling insecure... To not feel anxiety, that's what [that behaviour] stems from. (Ernest)

Men are a problem

In recent years, men have become a problem. That is, within many domains of life, relative to their female counterparts, men and boys are increasingly seen as somehow troubled or deficient. A slew of alarming statistics from the UK makes worrying reading. Take physical health. Life expectancy for men is currently 4.1 years lower than for women, with men more likely to die from the main common causes of death, such as cancer and heart disease (Office for National Statistics [ONS], 2012b). Or consider mental health. Men account for three-quarters of all suicide deaths (ONS, 2012d) and constitute 67 per cent of those detained in hospital under the Mental Health Act in England (NHS Information Centre, 2011). What about education? Boys are struggling at school, being outperformed by girls at all ages from 5 upwards, with 59 per cent of university entrants being female (Economic and Human Rights Commission [EHRC], 2011). Or crime? Men are more likely to commit and be the victim of violence, and overall constitute 95 per cent of the UK prison population (Ministry of Justice, 2012). Together, these figures paint a disturbing picture of a sex in trouble.

These types of figures should not imply that males are a subjugated gender, suffering while their female peers flourish. In many other respects, males overwhelmingly have the upper hand in terms of power or control, notwithstanding recent attempts to redress gender

1

imbalances. For example, at the start of 2013, men constituted 65 per cent of the senior civil service (ONS, 2011b), 77 per cent of FTSE 100 board members (Vinnicombe et al., 2010), 78 per cent of the judiciary (Judiciary of England and Wales, 2012), 78 per cent of MPs, 82 per cent of the Cabinet (www.parliament.co.uk, 2012), and 87 per cent of university heads (Universities UK, 2012). However, even though such figures appear to give men the 'upper hand', the performance of men here is still viewed as problematic. Male dominance in the public sphere is viewed as an issue to be rectified, and crucially, not simply because of the ideal of equality. For example, prominent financial writers have argued that with more females in positions of power, and less 'testosterone in the boardroom', recent financial crises could have been mitigated or even averted (Covert, 2012). Thus, men are still a problem.

However, even if there is a degree of consensus that men generally are a cause for concern, there are competing explanations for the causes of men's problems, and hence also for the solution to these. A prominent class of explanation adopts an essentialist perspective. Here, the attributes men are characterised as possessing – whether aggression, competitiveness or strength – are just the 'way men are'. One variety of this type of explanation is biological essentialism, which presents males as simply born that way. Take, for example, the above statistics pertaining to health. Beneath the bold headline mortality figure of men's lower life expectancy, subsequent details help to unpack this further. Men are more likely to die of the four most common causes of death, namely cancer, heart disease, respiratory diseases and cardiovascular diseases. At this point, it is tempting to agree with those biologists who argue that men are simply the weaker biological sex – 'nature's sole mistake' – burdened by a faulty Y chromosome that dooms them ineluctably to an early grave (Jones, 2003).

However, exploring men's poorer life expectancy further, the ONS then suggests that men's susceptibility to the common causes of death is partly due to 'lifestyle'. For example, men are more likely than women to be smokers (22 per cent of men vs. 18 per cent of women) and to binge drink (23 per cent vs. 14 per cent). These figures add to a growing body of work suggesting that men are prone to act in ways that have a detrimental impact upon their health. For example, men are seen as more likely to engage in 'health-risk' behaviours, such as illicit drug use (Farrell et al., 2001), dangerous driving (Lonczak et al., 2007) and unsafe sex (Flood, 2003). Men are also viewed as less willing to act in ways that would promote health, such as eating a healthy diet (Kiefer et al., 2005), seeking help for health problems (Galdas et al., 2005) or following treatment regimens (Obermeyer et al., 2004). Thus the argument shifts subtly from how men 'are' to how men 'act'.

With this shift, the type of explanation for the problem of men changes too. As the focus moves onto men's behaviour, there is conceptual space for explanations that consider the way this is shaped by social processes. That is not to say that biology might have no role to play in men's behaviour. For example, scholars continue to link testosterone – an androgen produced mainly in the testes, associated with secondary male sex characteristics such as facial hair – with behaviours viewed as typically male, such as aggression (Book et al., 2001) or risk-taking (Apicella et al., 2008). However, few scholars would endorse an extreme version of reductionism that positioned behaviour as entirely determined by biology. As such, to varying degrees, most thinking about men acknowledges that social factors have some influence on the way men behave. It is at this point that the argument about men, and whether they are indeed a problem, becomes interesting.

Variation in men

Until this point, I have used the word 'sex' to differentiate between men and women. It is generally acknowledged that categorising people as either male or female on the basis of agreed biological characteristics is standard practice in most societies, even if a minority of people defy easy categorisation (Brickell, 2006). However, in the 1950s, the term 'gender' came to prominence through the work of the sexologist John Money (Money et al., 1957). Thus in addition to the 'sex categories' of male and female, 'gender categories' of masculine and feminine entered the popular discourse. The nature of these different categories, and the relationships between them, is the subject of intense debate. However, as a useful starting point for conceptualising the difference between sex and gender, one could do worse than cite the World Health Organization [WHO] (2012). In their terms, sex refers to 'biological and physiological characteristics that define men and women'. In contrast, gender is 'the socially constructed roles, behaviours, activities, and attributes that a given society considers appropriate for men and women'.

With this distinction between sex and gender, it becomes apparent that the various problems associated with men are perhaps less about sex and more about gender. That is, if behaviours are shaped through social expectations and pressures around gender, our concern is not so much with men as with masculinity. So, for example, rather than men taking risks because of their biological sex status as males, we could understand such behaviour as the result of their feeling compelled to act this way because of what society expects from them 'as men'. This shift in perspective opens up some interesting possibilities. As the WHO suggests, while 'sex will not vary substantially between different human societies, aspects of gender may vary greatly'. And therein lies the hope for men, and the promise of this book. The idea that gender is not set in stone, that different societies can reach different conclusions for how men and women are or should be, means that the statistics cited above are not inevitable.

Thus, this book is part of an emergent body of work looking at variation in men, and in ideas around gender, i.e., societal expectations for how men *should* be. Such work is part of a larger current of poststructuralist thinking known as social constructionism. Such thinking does not simply contend that behaviour is shaped by social processes; after all, one can argue this, and yet still be susceptible to essentialism, seeing gender as a stable trait, fixed in childhood by socialisation pressures. Rather, the emphasis in social constructionism is very much on the word 'construction'. People are viewed as actively producing gendered selves through social interaction. So, for example, a man is not a risk-taker 'by nature', but takes risks in particular social situations because that is what he feels is expected of him. In this way, he defines himself as a man. Crucially, given the view above of men being 'a problem', social constructionist accounts of gender identify three important types of variation.

The first variation is perhaps easiest to recognise: there are differences among men, with all manner of shapes and sizes of personality. Thus, for example, even if men are more likely to binge drink than women, many men still avoid this kind of behaviour. The second variation is slightly harder to discern: there are differences *within* individual men, as behaviour changes according to the demands of particular social situations. That is, contrary to the 'trait' view of gender, individuals do not have a fixed character, but often alter their behaviour depending on circumstances. Thus a man might binge drink at a particular point in life, or around certain people, and then at other points, or with different people, find himself being more restrained. Finally, there is variation in terms of gender norms, i.e., 'roles, behaviours, activities, and attributes' deemed appropriate for men by a particular society. Crucially, this third variation contains many possibilities. It is not just that different cultures might have different expectations of men, e.g., different attitudes to drinking in Western and Islamic cultures. Cultures themselves can evolve, and also fragment, with gender norms shifting dynamically, in complex ways.

Intersecting ideas: Men are not necessarily a problem

So far, I have introduced two key ideas. The first is that 'men are a problem': men are encouraged by masculinity to behave in ways that are detrimental to health and wellbeing. However, the second idea is that there is variation in both men and masculinities. This book lies at the intersection of these two ideas. That is, deleterious 'traditional' masculine norms – e.g., toughness or risk-taking – are not inevitable. It is therefore possible that men can encounter and be influenced by 'positive' masculine norms, i.e., conducive to wellbeing. Thus my central aim is to explore the possibility that some men are able to take care of themselves, and engage 'constructively' with their wellbeing. In order to do this, the book draws on research conducted with a group of men who were considered likely to have found ways to skilfully manage their wellbeing. In particular, I chose to interview men who had taken up practising meditation. The reason for this choice will become apparent as the book proceeds. I was especially interested in hearing these men's narratives, that is, their stories about why they had decided to take up meditation, and how it had affected their lives.

By concentrating on men's narratives, I was able to get a sense of their journeys – as they told these at this particular point in their life – beginning in childhood, up until the time of their interview. These journeys illuminate many of the themes highlighted above: that boys and men are subject to socialisation pressures as they grow and develop; that these pressures can mean that males are encouraged or even compelled to act in ways that are detrimental to wellbeing; that gender is socially constructed, and as such, that it is possible for men to change their ways; and that some men can find more constructive means of engaging with their wellbeing. Moreover, by rooting the discussion of these ideas in the journeys of real men, rather than dealing in the currency of abstract concepts and dry statistical figures, this allows these ideas to come alive, to become more real and vivid to the reader. As such, apart from the first and last chapters, the book traces the journeys of these men, from childhood to the present day, interweaving theoretical ideas and empirical findings from the literature.

The book begins though with an opening chapter which outlines some of the key theoretical ideas that underpin subsequent chapters. These ideas fall into two main broad areas. Firstly, there is an introduction to some useful concepts relating to gender. For example, the book draws on work by Connell (1995) around the notion of 'hegemonic' masculinity. The idea is that there is variation both in men and in masculine norms, but that at any given time and place, a particular form of masculinity is valorised as *the* way to be a man. This idea helps explain why men can feel compelled to act in ways that may be detrimental to wellbeing. However, it also suggests that it is possible for new, more adaptive, norms to be fashioned. Secondly, the chapter gives a broad outline of a theory of wellbeing, which is conceived of as comprising multiple dimensions, including biological (e.g., physical health), psychological (e.g., happiness) and social dimensions (e.g., supportive relationships). This theory will be useful in exploring the various ways in which men both succeed and fail in promoting their own wellbeing. Finally, the chapter also says a little more about the research project that underpins the book, including how interviews were conducted and analysed.

The second chapter then begins to draw on the voices of the men I interviewed, using their narratives to illustrate and explore key ideas around masculinity and wellbeing. This chapter focuses on the start of their stories, beginning with their childhood and adolescence. Here we see how these men experienced pressure to be emotionally and physically tough, especially as they crossed a 'threshold' from boyhood to manhood, and felt sudden pressure to 'be a man'. This toughness had both outer and inner forms: participants learned to become hardened to people around them, and disconnected from their own emotions. The narratives highlight the weight of expectation upon boys as they are growing up, showing that traditional masculine norms play a significant role in shaping the way males engage with their interior world and with the world around them. It becomes clear that resisting 'traditional' hegemonic norms can be difficult, with implications for wellbeing. In particular, toughness norms meant men were often unwilling or unable to engage with their emotions – so-called 'restrictive emotionality' (Levant, 1992) – which meant men often had difficulties managing their emotions, leading to mental health issues in some cases.

In its largely 'negative' assessments of the detrimental impact of masculinity on wellbeing, the first chapter concurs with much of the literature in this area. However, the third chapter is where the book departs from this more common 'negative articulation' of masculinity, and brings in the idea of positive variation among men. Here, the focus is on how men managed to move away from their problematic behaviours and began to engage with their wellbeing by taking up meditation. Unfortunately though, this chapter shows that it often took something drastic to compel men to seek to change their ways, such as an emotional breakdown. Thus, the chapter echoes theoretical ideas around male depression, like Brownhill and colleagues' (2005) concept of the 'big build' – this involves escalating distress, featuring 'acting in' (emotional repression), culminating in 'acting out' crises, like a suicide attempt. Such crises finally compelled men here to take remedial action. That said, a minority of men found meditation in early adulthood, under less problematic circumstances. Their narratives thus offer useful clues about how the 'big build' might be circumvented.

The fourth chapter is where attention turns to meditation itself. At this point, it becomes clear why the research focused on meditators as potential exemplars of men who had found ways to engage with wellbeing. This chapter explores the idea that through meditation, men began to explore their 'inner world', thus moving away from the restrictive emotionality which had previously generated problems for them. Here I begin to outline a three-part model linking meditation to wellbeing: (a) meditation offered a system for training attention; (b) attention development helped improve men's emotional intelligence (EI); (c) enhanced EI facilitated wellbeing. This chapter focuses on (a), with (b) and (c) explored in Chapter 5. However, I also emphasise the gritty and often challenging process of learning meditation; this contrasts with much of the literature, which tends to present sanitised accounts glossing meditation in glowing terms as an easily-acquired panacea for all ills. For instance, men encountered troubling feelings in meditation which they sometimes lacked the skills to manage. Thus I strike a cautionary note of balance, showing that meditation is a powerful technique which needs to be respected as such, and taught/practised with caution.

Chapter 5 continues the exposition of the model linking meditation to wellbeing, outlining (b) and (c): attention development promoted EI, which then helped men engage constructively with their wellbeing. Men's accounts of developing EI aligned with Mayer and Salovey's (1997) hierarchical conceptual model of EI. That is, participants described acquiring, almost sequentially, skills of emotional awareness, generating emotions, emotional understanding and management of emotions. These EI skills were conducive to wellbeing both in and out of meditation. For example, in meditation, men were able to manage negative emotions through mental strategies, such as appraising negative qualia more dispassionately. Enhanced EI also meant men were more skilled at engaging with wellbeing in 'general life', outside meditation. For example, improved emotional understanding meant men were better able to resist urges to blunt their distress with alcohol, since they understood this would be counterproductive. Men also became better at engaging in health behaviours, partly due to experiencing greater self-control as a result of meditation. Social dimensions of wellbeing were also strengthened, as enhanced EI meant men were better at cultivating relationships.

The final chapter integrates the ideas from the previous chapters by outlining nine key 'lessons' from the book. These include practical recommendations for helping men to engage with their wellbeing through meditation. These recommendations are for professionals working with men (i.e., strategies to use with men), and for men themselves (i.e., 'self-administered' strategies). The first three lessons concern the need for men to engage with meditation in the first place, and ways in which this may be encouraged. The next four lessons pertain to meditation itself. Here, the chapter offers a stepwise series of practical exercises, structured to develop the four branches of EI in turn. Finally, the remaining two lessons offer practical guidance around helping men build, maintain and sustain a viable meditation practice in the context of their everyday masculine lives.

In sum, the book offers a message that is hopeful about the possibility of promoting positive changes in men, yet tempered with realism about the challenges of effecting these changes. In articulating and exploring this 'positive-yet-realistic' message, I have previously suggested that we are forging a new domain of scholarship, one I have referred to as 'critical positive masculinity' (Lomas, 2013). For those working with men, and for men themselves, I hope that you will find inspiration in the interviewees whose narratives form the substance of the book. I am grateful to have met these men, and to have heard their stories, and I am glad to be able to share these stories with you. These men's lives show that although learning to engage with wellbeing can be a hard road to take, it is a journey that is worth making.

1
Masculinity and Wellbeing

Blokes are terrible... Women are better about talking about feelings... maybe that's why women aren't on the whole so frustrated and angry about things. Men have got this big thing, 'No, we don't talk about that, get a beer, play some football, watch the football, buy a car, clean the car, anything but be with myself.' (Dean)

Setting the scene

This book will take you on a journey. We are going to trace the narratives of a group of men who appear to have found ways to positively engage with their wellbeing through meditation. Their stories will be used to illuminate a number of important ideas around masculinity and wellbeing. We will begin with stories from childhood and adolescence, showing how these men were influenced by masculine norms which encouraged them to be emotionally tough. We will see then how this toughness led them into difficulties, as they had a hard time coping with life, and with the negative emotions they suffered. We then move into more 'hopeful' territory, since these men were able to find better ways of engaging with their wellbeing by taking up meditation. Along the way, we will use these narratives to talk about key ideas and empirical findings that have emerged in the literature in recent years. By the end, I hope to have provided you with a detailed understanding of the complex connections between masculinity and wellbeing, and hopefully to also have offered a more optimistic prognosis for men.

Before embarking on this journey however, it is worth gathering some useful conceptual tools that will ease our subsequent passage. So, before introducing the men whose stories we shall be following, this first chapter introduces key theoretical ideas that will feature prominently in subsequent chapters. These ideas fall into two broad areas. First, I shall introduce concepts pertaining to gender. I will mention some more 'conventional' approaches to understanding gender, like gender stereotypes. I will then articulate a more dynamic social constructionist approach, which suggests gender is constantly being (re)created in the continual flux of social interaction. Second, I will articulate a multidimensional model for understanding wellbeing, featuring biological (e.g., physical health), psychological (e.g., mental health) and social dimensions (e.g., relational support). Subsequent chapters will then trace the intricate links between these two broad areas, i.e., the intersection between masculinity and wellbeing. Finally, the chapter ends by saying a little about the research that forms the basis of this book.

Gender

In trying to summarise the idea of gender, and masculinity in particular, one is assailed by a bewildering array of perspectives. Consequently, any book about masculinity, still less any chapter hoping to provide an introductory précis, cannot hope to be exhaustive. The best that can be hoped for is a sketch encompassing a number of key ideas, sufficient for articulating a coherent position on the topic. This, then, is the aim of this first section.

We begin by looking at the more conventional ways in which gender has been understood by academics – especially psychologists and sociologists – over recent decades. For instance, a large body of work on 'sex-differences' has articulated the notion that men and women act in different ways on account of their biologically-inherited predispositions. In contrast, other work on gender roles and stereotypes explores the influence of social learning, and the ways norms around masculinity help shape how men are raised and encouraged to behave. I then consider more recent social constructionist theorising which critiques the essentialism inherent in the more conventional approaches. Here, gender is viewed more as a performance constructed dynamically within social encounters. This view encourages the idea of gender as complex and fluid, capable of multiple forms of expression, and open to change. It is this more recent conceptualisation of gender which underpins the 'hopeful' message of this book.

Conventional approaches to gender

Among conventional approaches to gender, there are three main perspectives: biological, socio-cultural and psychological. We shall look at these in turn.

The biological perspective is the most straightforward. In essence, this conflates gender and sex: masculinity is simply how men are on account of their biological 'maleness'. This perspective is the one whose roots stretch back the farthest. It is here that we can locate the etymological origin of the term 'masculinity'. The Oxford English Dictionary [OED] (1971) suggests the word 'masculine' first came into use in the 14th century, via the Old French *masculin* (from the Latin *masculinus*, which itself was a diminutive of *mās*, meaning male). The term was initially used in a grammatical sense to denote the 'gender' of objects. However, by the 17th century it began to take on inflections suggesting qualities 'belonging' to males – the OED notes the use of masculine in 1629 to mean 'having the appropriate excellencies of the male sex: manly, virile, vigorous, powerful' (Masten, 1994). Such qualities had long been associated with men and manliness, featuring in some of the earliest works of literature, like the *Iliad* and the *Odyssey* from the 8th century BC (Van Nortwick, 2008). With the emergence of the term 'masculine' though, we find the beginnings of a subtle differentiation between men (sex), and qualities a culture expects them to possess (gender).

However, from the biological perspective, there is no meaningful separation between sex and gender. Gender is seen as the behavioural expression of biological attributes. Although this type of thinking has been strongly critiqued and found wanting – as explored below – it still finds voice in contemporary fields of academia, and society at large. This perspective often draws on ideas from evolutionary psychology to construct 'origin stories' about the historical emergence of particular gendered qualities (Eagly & Wood, 1999). For example, writers such as Geary (1998) argue that male promiscuity and aggression towards 'rivals' are behaviours that were 'selected for' in the evolutionary history of our species, as males exhibiting these qualities were more likely to propagate and pass on their genes. Academic research in this area is known as the 'sex-differences' paradigm (Maccoby & Jacklin, 1974), which analyses psychological and social outcomes on the basis of biological differences between the sexes.

Much of the sex-differences research on males concentrates on testosterone, an androgen produced mainly in the testes, associated with 'secondary male sex characteristics' such as facial hair (Wilhelm & Koopman, 2006). Numerous studies have linked testosterone levels to a range of behaviours viewed as typically male, including aggression (Book et al., 2001), risk-taking (Apicella et al., 2008), antisocial behaviour (Coren, 1998), competitiveness (Edwards et al., 2006) and even cognitive functions such as spatial abilities (O'Connor et al., 2001). In contrast, research on women often alights on the peptide hormone oxytocin, which is thought to underpin attachment behaviours (Neumann, 2008). As oxytocin is regulated by oestrogen, it is used to account for women's supposed nurturing tendencies (Campbell, 2008). This view of gender has considerable currency in society. For example, an emergent genre of discourse – labelled as 'neurosexism' by Fine (2008) – has latched selectively onto neuroscience research to portray men's and women's brains as 'hardwired' differently.

The biological determinism of the sex-differences approach has been roundly challenged by socio-cultural perspectives which suggest that gender is socially acquired. Conventional approaches here have focused on gender stereotypes and roles (sometimes referred to using the prefix 'sex' rather than gender). Gender stereotypes are 'beliefs about what it means to be male or female in terms of physical appearance, attitudes, interests, psychological traits, social relationships and occupations' (Granié, 2010, p. 727). Gender roles refer to the way particular behaviours and activities are not only encouraged as gender-appropriate on the basis of these stereotypes, but become institutionalised in the 'structural arrangements of a society' (West & Zimmerman, 1987, p. 128). It is argued that gendered behaviour emerges as stereotypes and roles are impressed upon children as they develop, with awareness of these emerging as early as 18 months old (Eichstedt et al., 2002). There are strong and weak versions of this argument. The weak version contends that biological predispositions linked to each sex are simply shaped by these socio-cultural forces. The strong version sees the child as a 'blank slate', with gender entirely the product of cultural conditioning.

While the strong version of this argument may be unpalatable to all but the most committed social constructionist, few people would deny that culture plays some role in fashioning our development as gendered beings. Various models have been articulated to understand this process of culturally influenced gender development. One prominent model is social learning theory (Mischel, 1975). This suggests that children observe and learn from the actions of significant others around them; these others also actively reinforce or discourage particular behaviours and qualities by rewarding or punishing them. Parents perhaps have the strongest influence in the earlier years; their beliefs about gender play a key role in shaping children's behaviour. For example, Morrongiello and Dawber (2000) examined how parental responses to the risk-taking behaviour of children differed according to sex, with parents more likely to intervene to prevent 'risky' play in girls, while tolerating or even encouraging it in boys. With age, other influences assume prominence, particularly peers (Hay et al., 1998), and prominent figures in the media (Witt, 2000). One driver of social learning is that self-esteem is linked to acceptance by others, which can be contingent on acquiescence to gendered norms (Smith & Leaper, 2006).

So, turning to masculine stereotypes in particular, what are some of the key ones that have been identified in contemporary 'Western' culture? Brannon (1976) identified four central stereotypes, which contemporary research has found are still influential. First is 'The big wheel', a concern with success and status. This is reflected in recent studies showing that people associate masculinity with dominance (de Pillis & de Pillis, 2008) or achievement (Jackson & Dempster, 2009). Second is 'Give 'em hell', where masculinity is identified with risk-taking behaviours, like alcohol use (de Visser et al., 2009), unsafe sex (Campbell, 1995) or dangerous driving (Schmid Mast et al., 2008), and with antisocial behaviour, from 'laddishness' (Francis, 1999) to violence (Moore & Stuart, 2005). Third is 'No sissy stuff', where qualities seen as 'feminine', like emotional expressiveness, are stigmatised and censured (Mejía, 2005). Lastly, 'The sturdy oak' valorises strength and toughness, with masculinity seen as epitomised by characteristics such as independence and self-reliance (Smith et al., 2007). A crucial aspect of the latter two stereotypes is emotional toughness – suppression, avoidance and reluctance or inability to express emotion (Cramer et al., 2005) – which plays a key role in later chapters.

While stereotypes refer to beliefs, roles reflect the way these beliefs create expectations that promote activities as gender-appropriate. For example, as noted above, endorsement of risk-taking stereotypes means parents are less likely to intervene to prevent risky play by boys (Morrongiello & Dawber, 2000). In this way, diverse spheres of activity – from sport (Tagg, 2008) to food consumption (Gough, 2007) – are regulated according to stereotypes which encourage/discourage participation on the basis of gender. Moreover, behaviours are not only encouraged, but institutionalised in societal structures, from implicit biases to explicit rules. Such institutionalisation is operative early in life. For instance, Anderson (2009, p. 4) argues that competitive sports are 'compulsory' for boys, reflecting sport's role as a potent vehicle for inculcating societies' 'gendered values, myths and prejudices'. In adulthood, gender roles are evident in gender-biases in employment, where the culture of certain jobs can be heavily gendered. For example, Thurnell-Read and Parker (2008, p. 127) describe the 'organisational structures, workplace practices and daily routines' of firefighting as 'steeped in maleness'. While the gendered composition of work is changing as women challenge prohibitive cultural and structural barriers (Kilminster et al., 2007), roles may still be reinforced through social pressure. This might include harassment of those who challenge convention, as witnessed recently with the first female beefeater (BBC, 2009).

Finally, some conventional theories understand gender from a psychological perspective. Here, the focus is on 'gender-identity', which refers to 'one's subjective sense of maleness/femaleness' (Kulis et al., 2008, p. 260). Theories here are often conceptualised using the stereotypes identified above; thus, gender-identity refers to the extent to which a person feels they adhere to these conventional stereotypes. For example, a popular assessment tool rates someone as having a masculine gender-identity if they identify themselves as being assertive (Bem, 1974). Interestingly, this perspective moves away from a strict male/female dichotomy. Masculinity and femininity are separate concepts rather than poles on a continuum, and people may feel they embody both masculine and feminine norms. This way of thinking has its roots in psychoanalytic theory. Freud (1918) wrote extensively about the complex internal structures of personality, for example. Through his intricate case studies, he was, as Connell (1995) acknowledges, a pioneer in the idea that 'masculine and feminine currents co-existed in everyone' (p. 9). Likewise, Jung (1951) argued that the psyche contained both a masculine (animus) and a feminine aspect (anima).

Some theories of gender-identity also focus on the extent to which people feel they *should* adhere to conventional stereotypes. For example, Pleck (1995) proposed the idea of gender role strain. Pleck argued that gender ideals can be hard to attain; e.g., men might struggle to be tough in the way that is expected. However, the psychological consequences of 'violating' gender expectations can be problematic. The theory has three components: (1) gender role discrepancy – differences between one's ideal and actual self can lower self-esteem; (2) gender role trauma – the socialisation processes through which fulfilment is encouraged can be traumatic, e.g., bullying; (3) gender role dysfunction – even if expectations are successfully met, this success may have negative consequences, since the desired behaviours can have a deleterious impact on wellbeing. This last item is a key theme of this book. For example, being tough may mean that men have difficulties managing their emotions. This last point is also reflected in O'Neil and colleagues' (1995) idea of 'gender role conflict'; this holds that people may be harmed by attempts to conform to gender norms, resulting in 'devaluation or violation of others or self' (p. 167).

Constructionist approaches to gender

Although many people still approach gender from these conventional perspectives, scholars working from a social constructionist standpoint have begun to articulate a more dynamic and nuanced reading of gender. Before exploring this in detail, it is worth saying something about social constructionism in general. Providing a concise summary of social constructionism is difficult since it is a 'broad church', incorporating diverse ideas and perspectives (Lock & Strong, 2010). Nevertheless, in this diversity, theorists recognise commonalities. Burr (1995) argues that various approaches share 'family resemblances', including preferences for anti-essentialism and anti-realism, recognition of the centrality of language in the production of knowledge, and awareness that our understanding of the world is historically and culturally situated. Constructionism is part of a broader current of thought known as poststructuralism. As Brickell (2005) explains, the former is a form of sociology, while the latter is a type of social theory, which has a much wider remit, encompassing 'all the disciplines concerned with the behaviour of human beings' (Giddens & Dallmayr, 1982, p. 5). Although poststructuralism is also hard to define, it can be understood by considering its predecessor, structuralism, from which it emerged as a critique (Marshall, 2010).

Structuralism originated in linguistics with de Saussure (1916). It proposed that phenomena derive meaning from their position within a network of other linguistic signs (Jenning, 1999). The concept of 'man', for example, only makes sense in relation to signifiers like 'woman'. However, while structuralism viewed language structures as largely fixed, poststructuralism recognised the shifting, dynamic nature of these structures (Marshall, 2010). Theorists such as Derrida (1982) argued that meaning is not unitary or fixed, but 'slippery and elusive' (Rail, 1998, p. xii), with multiple interpretations possible. Objects and categories of knowledge are not 'given by the world around us, but are instead produced by the symbolizing systems we learn' (Tyner, 2008, p. 4). As such, poststructuralism seeks to challenge terms 'that are assumed to be natural and unchanging', and to 'disrupt meaning, labels, and categories' (Tyner, 2008, p. 9). In this way, as a form of poststructuralism, social constructionism argues that concepts used to represent the world are socio-cultural products, reflecting 'historical and cultural understandings', rather than being 'universal and immutable categories of human experience' (Bohan, 1996, p. xvi).

The point about social constructionism is that it disrupts how we look at the world, showing that features or categories that we take to be 'natural' are created by social convention. For example, common sense suggests that sex categories – classifying people as male or female – are a fundamental distinction given by nature. However, constructionists argue that even these foundational distinctions are socially constructed. As the recent controversy around the South African runner Caster Semanya has shown – in a way that has been very challenging for the athlete herself – there is no empirical biological test to categorically assign a person to one sex or the other (Curley, 2012). As such, we classify people as male or female on the basis of socially agreed criteria, such as genitalia. However, this classification is arbitrary, and fails to account for those who do not fall neatly into either category (Lorber, 1996). Once this classificatory schema is operative though, it has a powerful normative force, structuring lives in 'profound ways', as most people are compelled to categorise themselves as either belonging to one sex or the other (Brickell, 2006, p. 100).

Compared to the sex categories of male and female, it is easier to see the gender categories of masculine and feminine as socially constructed. However, constructionist theorists still argue that the conventional approaches detailed above are guilty of essentialism, invoking 'singular categories of male and female' and presenting them as fixed 'containers' of stable attributes (Mac an Ghaill & Haywood, 2012, p. 483). This is reflected in the homogenising tendency towards making categorical generalisations about men or women as monolithic groups, e.g., ascribing definitive characteristics to *the* masculine personality. To take an example relevant to this book, it is often asserted that females are nearly twice as likely as men to experience depression. Although this book will critique this assertion – men may experience and express depression in ways not reflected in traditional diagnostic criteria (Kilmartin, 2005) – it is 'one of the most widely documented findings in psychiatric epidemiology' (Kessler, 2003, p. 6). In explaining this, Nolen-Hoeksema's (1987) influential 'sex-differences' theory suggested that these higher rates were due to women's different emotional responses: 'women's ruminative response styles amplify and prolong their depressive episodes... [whereas] men's active response styles dampen their depressive episodes' (p. 276).

It is not only biological approaches to gender that are subject to essentialism. Even theories that recognise the influence of culture, like social learning theories, are usually essentialist, viewing gender as 'fixed, unvarying and static – much like sex' (West & Zimmerman, 1987, p. 126). For example, over time, Nolen-Hoeksema's theory has evolved from 'Sex differences in unipolar depression' (1987) to 'Gender differences in depression' (2001). However, the latter still made categorical generalisations, such as 'gender differences in rumination at least partly account for the gender differences in depression' (p. 175). Thus, although the discourse had shifted to socially-produced gender patterns, the tendency to essentialise the differences between men and women remained. However, in contrast to these conventional approaches, emergent constructionist theories of gender emphasise agentic *construction*. Here, people are not regarded as 'passive victims of a socially prescribed role', nor 'simply conditioned or socialised by their cultures', but as 'active agents', continually engaged in constructing gender in their interactions (Courtenay, 2000, pp. 1387–1388).

Viewing people as actively engaged in an on-going project of gender construction introduces two key ideas: the concept of 'doing' gender (West & Zimmerman, 1987), and the diversity of gender constructions (Connell, 1995). First, in terms of 'doing' gender, constructionist theories of identity move away from the essentialist idea of gender as a static psychological property or trait – even if learned through socialisation – towards a 'process' orientated view (Lorber, 1996). Gender is not seen as a fixed attribute, located 'within' the individual, but a fluid process, generated by the dynamics of social interaction. West and Zimmerman (1987, p. 140) captured this shift in perspective from attribute to process by arguing that gender should be seen more as a verb than a noun: rather than something one 'has' or 'is', gender is 'something one does, and does recurrently, in interaction with others'.

From this dynamic constructionist perspective, gender is seen in relational terms as a product of social interaction – as 'a set of socially constructed relationships which are produced and reproduced through people's actions' (Gerson & Peiss, 1985, p. 327). This contrasts with the way conventional theories generally view gender in individual terms as a personal attribute. Moreover, gender is a dynamically evolving process, not a static, stable configuration. People are seen as continually engaged in constructing/re-constructing their gendered identity as they negotiate their social world (McKinlay, 2010). The idea of understanding gender in relational terms derives from structuralism (Lévi-Strauss, 1981). However, it is the emphasis on the fluid nature of these social productions – i.e., that gender is 'not static but rather is constantly (re)defined and contested in the contexts within which it is invoked' (Nightingale, 2006, p. 171) – that marks these theories as poststructuralist.

This process-oriented view of gender was captured persuasively by Butler (1990), with her influential notion of performativity. Butler argued that people do not have a foundational gendered identity generating their actions in a causal way – e.g., risk-taking *because* they are masculine – no 'ontological subject that prefigures action' (Nayak & Kehily, 2006, p. 460). Instead, gender is produced through one's actions: one becomes masculine by taking risks. Rejecting essentialist notions of self, Butler draws on Nietzsche's idea of there being 'no doer behind the deed' (Digeser, 1994). Gendered identity is thus seen as the effect, not the cause, of a person's repeated behaviours: 'Repetition is not performed *by* a subject; this repetition is what enables a subject' (Butler, 1993, p. 95). This lack of a 'doer' raises the question of who or what *is* the cause of such behaviour, if not the person themselves. Here, it is argued that the repetition of particular behaviours is policed by 'regulatory regimes', i.e., social pressures which encourage a 'forced reiteration of norms' (McKinlay, 2010, p. 235). Thus, although there is no essential masculinity, regulatory regimes enforce the persistence of traditional gender behaviours (the roles and stereotypes discussed above).

A similar explanation for the persistence of traditional gender behaviour is found in Connell's (1995) influential theory of masculinities. This brings us to the second key idea introduced by constructionist theories: the diversity of gender constructions. Connell shifted the focus from singular masculinity to masculini*ties*, drawing attention to the variety of forms of masculinity enacted in everyday practices. However, in a given context, a particular form of masculinity – the 'most honored way of being a man' (Connell & Messerschmidt, 2005, p. 832) – becomes normative. This dominant form is called 'hegemonic masculinity'. The concept of hegemony was adapted from Gramsci (1971), who argued that societal inequalities are entrenched since people in power maintain control not only via political dominance, but more assiduously via ideological influence which legitimises the status quo. Connell argued that masculinities exist in hierarchical relationships, with a particular form of behaviour culturally authoritative in a given setting. Hegemonic masculinity dominates subordinate and marginalised masculinities through a normalising ability to frame behaviours as natural, and an ability to levy penalties on those who deviate from expectations (Moss-Racusin et al., 2010). An example here is the way homosexuality, usually viewed as a marginalised masculinity, is 'censured' (Roberts, 1993), from bullying to anti-gay violence (Mills et al., 2004).

To the extent that Connell recognised that certain forms of masculinity become dominant, he is in accord with the conventional notions of gender roles and stereotypes. However, he also emphasised that the dominant forms varied according to context. Rejecting static ideas of *the* masculine stereotype, he argued that local milieus valorised particular masculinity forms as hegemonic. Thus, different forms of gendered behaviour – 'configurations of practice that are accomplished in social action' (Connell & Messerschmidt, 2005, p. 836) – emerge in different contexts. This idea is reinforced by research examining variance in actual hegemonic forms. For example, studying the Norwegian logging industry, Brandth and Haugen (2005) found that hegemonic norms included the possession of a 'weathered' countenance, reflecting years of outdoor toil. Moreover, hegemonic norms shifted over time, even in this narrow context, as changes to working practices meant that ability to wield heavy machinery had since become valorised. Comparable diversity among hegemonic forms has been studied at varying levels of scale. Cross-cultural analyses show national-level variations, from Argentinean machismo (Stobbe, 2005) to a post-conflict nationalistic Kosovan masculinity (Munn, 2008). More specific groups or locales studied include the US Navy (Barrett, 1996), working-class youth in post-industrial northern England (Nayak, 2006), 'transnational' business executives (Connell & Wood, 2005) and netball players in New Zealand (Tagg, 2008).

Theorists have sought to understand how local contexts can promote particular formations of gendered behaviour. Some have used Lave and Wenger's (1991) concept of communities of practice (CoP) as a framework for analysing how identities are learned and reproduced in social groups (Creighton, 2011). Although CoP is an evolving and contested concept (Lindkvist, 2005), a good definition is 'people who come together around mutual engagement in an endeavour' and the practices which 'emerge in the course of this' (Eckert & McConnell-Ginet, 1992, p. 464). In terms of masculinity, Paechter (2003, p. 72) argues that CoP enable the 'production, reproduction, and negotiation' of particular forms of gendered behaviour by encouraging such behaviour as a condition of participation, and eventually 'full membership', in the group.

Most studies have emphasised the role of CoP in the maintenance of traditional masculine norms. For example, Parker (2006) studied how the 'occupational culture' of a football team socialised its members into adopting 'stereotypical' masculine behaviours. However, it is not inevitable that CoP promote 'traditional' norms. Golding and colleagues (2008) examined the Australian 'shed' movement, a network of informal 'workshop-based spaces' that give men an opportunity to socialise and share skills. These CoP offered a 'safe space' that allowed the emergence of 'non-traditional qualities' in men, such as emotional expression.

The possibility that CoP can promote alternative 'positive hegemonic masculinities' – ones that are more conducive to wellbeing – will be returned to in later chapters when we consider the social dimensions of meditation practice.

The idea that specific contexts encourage particular forms of behaviour has some important consequences. In particular, this means there is not only diversity among men, but *within* individual men. Connell's theory does not simply describe a 'typology' of men, making the rather obvious point that different men have different characters and personalities (although some critics accused the theory of doing this, notably Wetherell and Edley (1999)). Rejecting essentialism, the theory makes the more radical point that men take up different subject positions according to need. Various enactments of masculinity represent not different types of men, but reflect how men strategically 'position themselves through discursive practices' according to the dynamics of the social situation (Connell & Messerschmidt, 2005, p. 841). As Paechter (2003, p. 69) put it, this means a 'multiplicity of masculinities, inhabited and enacted by different people and by the same people at different times'. This view of gender has challenging implications for the idea of identity. The self is viewed as the site of confluence for competing masculine discourses of masculinity. This view reflects poststructuralist conceptions of identity, which reject the idea of a singular, coherent, unified and autonomous self. Instead, the self is seen as a multiplicity of competing and overlapping voices, urges, ideas, beliefs and feelings (Gergen, 2001).

However, although there is no unitary self in this view, Connell and Messerschmidt (2005, p. 843) contend that this does not 'erase the subject'. There is still a place here for agency and subjectivity, a volitional self who acts and experiences. They reject 'structural determinism', the idea that behaviour is inextricably conditioned by one's context. In their view, men do have some freedom in the type of gendered performance they enact. However, this freedom is 'constrained massively' by various factors, 'by embodiment, by institutional histories, by economic forces, and by social and family relationships' (p. 843). In particular, men are constrained by hegemonic masculinity. Thus, although masculinity is socially constructed, and multiple masculinities are acknowledged, as with Butler's regulatory regimes, hegemony explains why particular forms of masculinity nevertheless become dominant.

As such, while hegemonic masculinity may not be a statistical norm – only a minority may successfully enact it – it is normative. From this perspective, the stereotypes outlined above can be understood as 'traditional' hegemonic norms which men feel pressured to enact, or else resist at the risk of censure. The key idea, one that is central to this book, is that such norms may be detrimental to wellbeing. Throughout the chapters, our focus will be on the ways in which hegemonic masculinity intersects with wellbeing – how traditional norms might hinder wellbeing, and how men can perhaps find more constructive ways of 'doing' masculinity. However, before starting on this journey, we also need to articulate a basic model of wellbeing. This is outlined next.

Wellbeing

Over recent years, the term 'wellbeing' has become increasingly visible in modern society. We see it used enthusiastically, often in conjunction with the word 'health', in a bewildering variety of contexts, from academic literature to government policy documents to advertising campaigns. Despite this prominence however, its precise meaning is slippery and vague. Of course, from a social constructionist perspective, all words are conceptually indeterminate – their meaning is contestable, open to multiple interpretations, and subject to change (Derrida, 1982). Naturally, wellbeing is no different. As de Chavez and colleagues (2005) elucidate, the term is used in diverse ways by different theoretical frameworks, as will be outlined below. For example, some psychological models focus on positive mood, while biomedical conceptualisations tend to equate wellbeing with physical health. Given the range of uses for which the term has been put to work, it can be difficult to get a clear conceptual grasp of this important idea. However, help is at hand from a model developed first within medicine.

The biopsychosocial model was proposed by Engel (1977) as a 'holistic' approach to health. He hoped this would supersede the more reductive 'medical model' of disease, which tended to focus just on body dysfunction. Beyond the physical illness, Engel also sought to account for 'the patient, the social context in which he lives, and the complementary system devised by society to deal with the disruptive effects of illness' (p. 132). The model is slowly gaining acceptance within medicine, becoming incorporated into training and practice (Adler, 2009). Moreover, the idea of a biopsychosocial approach has become increasingly influential in other contexts. De Chavez and colleagues argue that there is an increasing trend in academia and beyond for articulating a multidimensional approach to wellbeing. For example, Pollard and Davidson (2001, p. 10) define wellbeing as 'a state of successful performance throughout the life course integrating physical, cognitive and social-emotional function'. Thus, we can view wellbeing as comprising physical, psychological and social dimensions. Keeping in mind that wellbeing is a function of *all* these dimensions, we can explore them in turn here to get a clearer sense of the different aspects of wellbeing.

Physical dimensions of wellbeing

When we talk about the physical dimensions of wellbeing, we are generally referring to the idea of 'health'. The conceptual relationship between health and wellbeing is interesting. Sometimes these terms are used somewhat synonymously, sometimes wellbeing is seen as a component of health, and sometimes health is viewed as an aspect of wellbeing. Larson (1999) outlines four different models of health, encompassing all these different uses: the 'WHO model'; the 'wellness model'; the 'medical model'; and the 'environmental model'. We will consider these briefly, before suggesting that we can arrive at an understanding of health that draws on all four models. However, following de Chavez et al. (2005), I will then argue that we should view health as just one dimension of a broader idea of wellbeing.

The WHO's widely cited definition of health is unchanged since 1948: 'a state of complete physical, mental and social well-being and not merely the absence of disease and infirmity' (WHO, 1948). Here, health is viewed as a polarity, with wellbeing its positive pole, illness its negative. In contrast, the wellness model uses health and wellbeing synonymously. This approach is less concerned with alleviating illness, focusing more on attaining 'higher levels of health and wellness' (Larson, 1999, p. 128). In the reductive 'medical model' of health, there is little mention of wellbeing. The individual is seen in mechanical terms as a system of parts: disease is a 'dysfunction of the body', and health the absence of dysfunction (Patel et al., 2002, p. 8). While this model has formed the basis of modern Western medical approaches, it has been criticised as dehumanising, reducing people to component parts and ceding control over the body to health professionals (Frank, 1997). Finally, the environmental model concerns successful adaptation to one's environment. In contrast to the medical model, here the individual is seen as a volitional agent, sharing responsibility for their health through behaviour. This last perspective informs much health promotion literature, such as efforts to encourage people to exercise (Simon et al., 2009).

Thus, there are different conceptualisations of health. However, we can sensibly arrive at an understanding of health that incorporates ideas from all the models. For example, as per the medical model, we can agree that health includes (relative) freedom from dysfunction and disease. At the same time, following the environmental model, we can appreciate the role that people can play in fostering their own physical health through their actions. We can identify behaviours which constitute a healthy lifestyle, including maintaining a programme of regular exercise, a balanced diet, good sleep habits, and refraining from excessive alcohol and tobacco consumption (Danna & Griffin, 1999). Moreover, these behaviours may not only help to prevent illness, they can also encourage higher degrees of health and physical functioning (beyond just freedom from disease), which resonates with the wellness model.

Health is viewed as a substantive good – we value it for its own sake. However, we can also appreciate health as an instrumental good, since it impacts upon the other dimensions of wellbeing. Here we can appreciate the way these different dimensions of wellbeing are interrelated. For example, satisfaction with life is one element of the psychological dimension of wellbeing, as set out below. As one can perhaps expect, life satisfaction is adversely affected by illness (Breitbart et al., 2000) and disability (Uppal, 2006). However, as we shall see, such conditions have less of an impact on wellbeing than might be anticipated, as people generally adapt well, usually within a few months (Lee et al., 2000). Conversely, in terms of health behaviours, exercise is not only health promoting, it is also associated with life satisfaction (Reed & Ones, 2006). However, it is also important to see health as just one aspect of a broader concept of wellbeing, i.e., its physical aspect. We now move on to the psychological dimensions of wellbeing.

Psychological dimensions of wellbeing

From a psychological perspective, wellbeing can either be conceptualised negatively as the absence of mental illness and distress, or positively as the presence of desiderata, such as pleasure (Hatch et al., 2010). Historically, psychology has generally sought to emulate the medical model of health, pursuing a 'negative' approach to wellbeing (Ryff & Singer, 1998). The focus has tended to be on psychological dysfunction, and how this might be ameliorated. This perspective is encapsulated by Freud's (in)famous remark (to a hypothetical patient) that psychotherapy could aim no higher than hoping to transform the misery of neurosis into 'common unhappiness' (Breuer & Freud, 1893–1895/1955, p. 305). However, a recent countermovement has emerged in the shape of 'positive psychology', which seeks to articulate wellbeing in more 'positive terms' (Seligman & Csikszentmihalyi, 2000). Positive psychology defines itself as a 'science that strives to promote flourishing and fulfillment' (Linley & Joseph, 2004, p. xv). We will see that both the negative and positive perspectives will be useful in subsequent chapters.

The negative perspective

Taking first the 'negative' perspective, wellbeing is the (relative) absence of mental illness and distress. Mental illness refers to discrete illness categories defined by the *Diagnostic and Statistical Manual of Mental Disorders* (DSM-V; American Psychiatric Association [APA], 2013). The most common disorders are depression and anxiety (Kessler et al., 2005). Depression refers to a spectrum of mood disturbance (mild to severe, transient to persistent). Its cardinal symptoms are low mood and diminished interest in pleasure. Major depressive disorder is diagnosed if five or more symptoms persist over a two-week period. Subtypes include bipolar (alternating with mania) and adjustment disorders (resulting from stressful events). Anxiety is also on a continuum, from mild (which can be adaptive, e.g., as a warning signal), to severe (interferes with functioning). It has various subtypes, including generalised anxiety disorder (unfocused worry), social anxiety disorder (fear of social situations), panic disorder, and specific phobias.

Although depression and anxiety are considered separate, they often co-occur, and thus are referred to as common mental disorders (CMDs; Goldberg & Huxley, 1992). CMDs involve a mix of anxiety and depressive symptoms, and are mental conditions that cause 'appreciable emotional distress and interfere with daily function', as McManus and colleagues (2009, p. 11) put it. Finally, in contrast to identified disorders, distress is more general in definition and measurement, with symptoms not specific to particular disorders (Marchand et al., 2005). Distress denotes negative experiences that fall short of clinical diagnoses for disorders, though there may be overlap; it can range from 'normal' levels of negativity, to levels approaching clinical significance that fulfil diagnostic criteria for depression and anxiety (Green et al., 2010). I should note that some of these definitions will be critiqued in later chapters, since we will explore the possibility that men may experience depression in ways not covered by generic diagnostic criteria. Nevertheless, as an initial sketch of some of the key concepts in mental health, the foregoing will suffice.

Before moving on to the positive perspective, it is pertinent to introduce a number of concepts relating to mental illness that will be useful in later chapters. While there are a variety of different theoretical frameworks for understanding mental illness and distress, two will be particularly relevant here. The first is the cognitive approach, which explains mental illness in terms of dysfunctional mental processes. Within this approach, some theories have alighted on attentional information-processing biases. For example, depression is linked to selective preferences for attending to negative stimuli (Strunk & Adler, 2009). Other cognitive theories focus on maladaptive thought patterns, as reflected in cognitive therapy (Beck et al., 1979). Depression is seen as linked to a dysfunctional 'triad' of thought patterns, an attribution style which interprets negative events as internal (self-caused), stable (linked to enduring factors) and global (universally applicable); thus, a response to failure might be, 'I'm always bad at everything' (Abramson et al., 1978). Depression is also associated with rumination, i.e., 'repetitively thinking about the causes, consequences and symptoms of one's negative affect' (Smith & Alloy, 2009, p. 117). Cognitive therapy aims to challenge and reconfigure these 'depressogenic' thought patterns.

A second important theoretical framework is the 'psychosocial stressors' perspective. This takes a broad view encompassing psychological and social factors, emphasising that stressful life events can precipitate mental health issues, particularly anxiety and depression (Tennant, 2002). As Turner and Lloyd (2004, p. 481) put it, adversity is 'causally implicated in the onset of depressive and anxiety disorders'. However, the issue is not just 'exposure' to stressors: people differ in their ability to cope. It is recognised that particular events are inherently stressful, the most potent being – in order – the death of a spouse or child, divorce, death of a family member, marital separation, becoming unemployed, and major personal injury/illness (Holmes & Rahe, 1967; Scully et al., 2000). However, recognising that many of these events are perhaps unavoidable in the long run, research has focused on people's ability to cope with such events.

Theorists have suggested that stress occurs when the demands imposed on an individual by their environment exceed their ability to cope (Lazarus & Folkman, 1987). However, people differ in how they try to cope with stress. Theorists have identified various coping strategies, or 'response styles' (Carver et al., 1989). These are classified as 'problem-focused' (targeting the stressor), 'emotion-focused' (managing reaction to the stressor), or 'avoidance-focused' (escaping the problem). These strategies can also be either cognitive or behavioural. A cognitive problem-focused response could be rumination (Nolen-Hoeksema, 1991), while a behavioural response could be 'confronting' the problem (Kaiseler et al., 2009). Emotion-focused cognitive responses include cultivating positive thoughts (Luginaah et al., 2002), and behavioural responses may involve expressing one's feelings (Stanton et al., 2000).

With avoidance, a cognitive response may be distracting oneself from the stressor (Appelhans et al., 2011), while behavioural responses include suppressing negative thoughts through psychoactive substances (Benson, 2010), or avoidance of situations featuring the stressor (Plexico et al., 2009).

Crucially, different strategies are usually categorised as being adaptive (alleviating distress, and protective against disorders) or maladaptive (exacerbating distress, and implicated in disorders) (Aldao et al., 2010). The most maladaptive strategies are rumination and avoidance. Rumination is seen as a dysfunctional cognitive style that contributes to depression, drawing people into a 'downward' spiral of negative thoughts and worsening negative affect (Teasdale et al., 2000). Avoidance is causally linked to numerous disorders, including anxiety (Roemer & Borkovec, 1994), depression (Borton et al., 2005), panic (Spira et al., 2004) and self-harm (Chapman et al., 2005). Avoidance is counterproductive since not only are attempts to suppress thoughts and emotions ineffectual, this actually increases the salience of suppressed qualia, exacerbating distress (Wegner & Gold, 1995). Moreover, by not engaging with either the stressor or with one's emotional reaction to it, there is a danger that the problem will build until it culminates in a destructive way, like an emotional breakdown (Brownhill et al., 2005). Significantly, men are seen as more likely to engage in avoidance coping responses (Aldao et al., 2010). We shall have much more to say about this in Chapter 3.

While rumination and avoidance are viewed as counterproductive, from a larger perspective these responses are indicative of a more general issue of emotional management. The concept of emotional management has been developed across various models, including emotion work (Ainsworth et al., 1979), emotional regulation (Gross, 1999) and emotional intelligence (Mayer & Salovey, 1997). These models are located within a wider framework of self-regulation theory, encompassing regulation of motivation, cognition, social interactions and behaviour (Carver & Scheier, 1998). Here, individuals are seen as volitional agents, capable of goal selection, decision making, planning and goal-directed determination. In this context, emotional management concerns the self-regulation of emotion, using cognitive and behavioural strategies to evoke, suppress or alter feelings and emotions. The goal of these strategies is to reduce negative affect through the selection and implementation of specific coping strategies. It is argued that *inability* to manage one's emotions is a crucial factor underlying diverse mental health conditions (Aldao et al., 2010).

As we shall see, the idea of emotional management will be central to this book. To give a brief preview of how: it is argued that masculine norms around emotional toughness mean that men are liable to have particular difficulties with emotional management (Addis, 2008). Consequently, men may have difficulties dealing with stress and distress, frequently turning to 'maladaptive' avoidant coping strategies, such as blunting with alcohol. However, it appears that meditation is one way in which men can improve their emotional management skills, and hence engage with their wellbeing, as the second half of the book explores.

Now I shall continue to outline a general model of wellbeing, turning to the 'positive' aspects of the psychological dimension.

The positive perspective

The negative perspective focuses on psychological phenomena that prevent wellbeing, such as mental illness. In contrast, the new 'positive psychology' movement that has emerged in recent years has sought to identify the psychological qualities and attributes we should *strive towards* in our pursuit of wellbeing. This movement was inaugurated only as recently as 1998, when Martin Seligman was elected to the presidency of the American Psychological Association (Fowler et al., 1999). Many of the ideas explored by positive psychology are not new; in fact, the strength of the movement lies in the way it brought together a diverse range of ideas under one banner. These ideas were drawn from various schools of thought, not only psychology, but religion, philosophy, economics and politics. While there is naturally a wide spectrum of ideas within the field of positive psychology, scholars distinguish between three main 'types' of wellbeing: subjective wellbeing (SWB), psychological wellbeing (PWB) and engaged wellbeing (EWB).

The idea of SWB – sometimes called *hedonic* wellbeing – is rooted in utilitarian notions of happiness (Diener & Oishi, 2000). This notion has a proud history in the writings of scholars such as Bentham (1776), who argued that we should seek 'the greatest happiness for the greatest number', but did not necessarily distinguish between different *types* of happiness.

Current conceptualisations of SWB view it as composed of two components: affective and cognitive. Affect – encompassing mood and emotion – comprises negative affect (NA) and positive affect (PA) (Diener & Emmons, 1984). Although these are orthogonal constructs, subjectively they represent a single dimension: we cannot feel both simultaneously, and each dampens the other (Green & Salovey, 1999).

In addition, orthogonal to PA and NA is an arousal axis, thus PA may be aroused (joy) or un-aroused (contentment) to various degrees, while NA may be aroused (anxious) or un-aroused (depressed) to various degrees (Russell et al., 1989). Self-reported levels of affective SWB reflect the balance, or 'ratio', of PA and NA. The cognitive component of SWB refers to judgements of life satisfaction, representing a 'global assessment of a person's quality of life according to his [sic] chosen criteria' (Shin & Johnson, 1978, p. 478). While ratings of affective SWB are more reflective of relatively short-term situation-dependent feelings of mood, cognitive SWB derives from more stable longer-term evaluations (Pittau et al., 2010).

A key issue in positive psychology is around the extent to which SWB is amenable to change (i.e., are efforts to enhance our happiness in vain?). Theories of SWB construct it as relatively stable over time and circumstance. 'Set-point' theory proposes that SWB levels fluctuate around a stable set-point, determined largely by genetic factors, which account for about 50 per cent of the variance in SWB (Lykken & Tellegen, 1996). A related theory is the hedonic treadmill (Brickman & Campbell, 1971). This argues that losses or gains in SWB due to circumstantial changes are temporary, as people adapt and revert to their 'set-point', usually within three months (Suh et al., 1996). These theories were prompted by striking studies which suggested that positive events like winning the lottery did not raise SWB long-term (Brickman et al., 1978), while negative events like spinal injury did not seem to significantly lower it (Chwalisz et al., 1988). However, other work suggests that some events may leave such emotional scarring as to permanently lower SWB, like the death of a child (Wortman & Silver, 1989) or repeated long-term unemployment (Lucas et al., 2004). Conversely, longitudinal studies have also found permanent increases in SWB, for example in people who become more religious over time (Headey et al., 2010).

As such, refinements to hedonic theory suggest set-levels can be altered. To account for the possibility of altering SWB, Lyubomirsky and colleagues (2005) have proposed a dynamic theory of wellbeing comprising three determinants: genetic set-point; circumstances; and activities. As noted, genetic inheritance accounts for about 50 per cent of the variance in SWB. Lyubomirsky estimated that 10 per cent of the variance is thus determined by our circumstances, and 40 per cent by intentional activities. I shall say more about circumstantial factors when we consider the social dimensions of wellbeing below. Suffice to say that the World Values Survey, charting the SWB of over 87,000 people across 46 countries, found the four most important factors were: marriage, financial situation, work, and friends and community (Helliwell & Putnam, 2004). It appears our best hope of raising our SWB lies with intentional activities. On-going efforts to engage in practices that promote wellbeing have a cumulative impact that leads to durable increases in SWB. These practices could be behavioural (e.g., exercise), cognitive (e.g., meditation) or 'volitional' (e.g., striving towards a cause). We will see that meditation is a particularly potent intentional activity, with implications for SWB.

While SWB focuses on pleasure and satisfaction, psychological wellbeing (PWB) is subtly different. PWB is often referred to as *eudaimonic* wellbeing, a term derived from Aristotle pertaining to human 'flourishing' (translated literally as 'good spirit'). In our contemporary language, 'flourishing' is recast as 'optimal functioning', and is described as 'committing oneself to a meaningful and purposeful life' (Keyes et al., 2002, p. 1018). While SWB only concerns the *amount* of happiness one experiences, PWB involves the value judgement that some types of activities and attributes are *qualitatively better* than others, more fulfilling and rewarding. More contentiously, PWB theory suggests that people who engage in these activities and possess these attributes are more 'developed' and have a greater worth. This viewpoint was famously expressed by Mill (1863, p. 9), who argued that it was 'better to be Socrates dissatisfied than a fool satisfied'. PWB has its roots in two traditions of thought that were prominent in the 20th century: existentialism and humanism. From these sources, positive psychology has identified various features of a 'purposeful and meaningful' life.

Existentialism is a disparate body of thought whose common point of reference is analysis of the 'human condition' (Yalom, 1980). Emerging in the 19th century with Kierkegaard (1843) and Nietzsche (1886), it flourished in post-World War II Europe with writers such as Camus (1942) and Sartre (1943). Existentialism focuses on common themes seen as inescapable features of human existence, the 'ultimate concerns' of life. Foremost among these is the idea that it is incumbent upon people to find meaning – especially since the erosion of religious belief has denuded the world of any intrinsic meaning – or else suffer despair (Tillich, 1952). In seeking meaning, we need both comprehensibility (making sense of life) and significance (endowing it with purpose) (Janoff-Bulman & Yopyk, 2004). Here existentialists emphasise the 'burden' of freedom (Heidegger, 1927). The burden is threefold. First, we must take responsibility for choices, even as these are constrained by contingencies (i.e., we find ourselves 'thrown' into situations not of our own making). Second, we must strive for authenticity, not 'flee' this burden and allow one's goals to be determined by others. Finally, we need to be resolute and pursue meaning despite knowing that it is ultimately futile in the face of one's eventual death.

A second school of thought which gave rise to the notion of PWB was humanism. From here came the idea that, in addition to living a meaningful life, wellbeing meant striving to realise one's potential to 'use and develop the best in oneself' (Huta & Ryan, 2010, p. 735). In this respect, positive psychology drew on humanistic notions of the possibility of psychological development across the lifespan (Resnick et al., 2001). For example, Rogers (1951), the pioneer of humanistic psychotherapy, articulated a view of therapy as a process of helping to bring 'inner' potentialities to realisation. From one perspective, this idea of growth can be interpreted as helping people lead more 'authentic' lives – finding out their particular strengths and structuring their lives around these (Seligman et al., 2005). From another perspective, this idea can assume a hierarchical inflection, as people are seen as being at different developmental stages (Linley & Joseph, 2004). This draws on theorists who have articulated structural developmental schemas for various capacities, like values (Graves, 1970), morals (Kohlberg, 1968) and needs (Maslow, 1943). PWB is thus seen as reflecting the attainment of higher 'stages' of development in these capacities.

Drawing on these schools of thought, theorists have proposed various models of PWB. Ryff and Keyes' (1995) PWB theory identifies six key components that are central to PWB: autonomy, purpose in life, personal growth, positive relations, environmental mastery and self-acceptance. A similar model, which also encompasses motivation and values, is Ryan and Deci's (2000) self-determination theory. This holds that people's 'innate' tendencies towards growth are promoted or thwarted depending on whether they are allowed to satisfy three basic psychological needs: competence (exercising their abilities), relatedness (interpersonal connectedness) and autonomy (freedom and choice). In addition to the meeting of these needs, two other factors central to PWB: being mindful (acting with awareness) and pursuing intrinsic rather than extrinsic goals (Ryan et al., 2008). This last point is interesting. PWB is not just about people having self-determination to pursue goals that are personally important (intrinsically motivated), rather than imposed on them by others through rewards or punishment (extrinsically motivated). This theory also suggests that some goals and values are 'intrinsically' better than others.

It is here that theorists begin to talk about values. Some values are seen as more conducive to PWB than others. As a point of contrast, we can highlight two sets of values seen as having opposing effects upon wellbeing. On one hand, materialism – 'centrally held beliefs about the importance of possessions in one's life' (Richins & Dawson, 1992, p. 308) – is generally seen as a value that is not conducive to wellbeing (Roberts & Clement, 2007). One explanation is that material acquisitions are particularly susceptible to 'adaptation', as per the idea of the hedonic treadmill (Chancellor & Lyubomirsky, 2011). Unfortunately, materialism is arguably the dominant ideology of late modernity; Carlisle and colleagues (2009) have thus suggested that wellbeing is a 'collateral causality' of our present consumer society. In contrast, the pursuit of values associated with religion is seen as conducive to PWB, especially values relating to personal relationships. PWB is linked to the expression of qualities like altruism (Borgonovi, 2008), forgiveness (Lawler-Row, 2010), compassion (Gilbert, 2005), gratitude (Wood et al., 2008) and trust (Soroka et al., 2003). While one can of course pursue these qualities without being religious, religions are seen as particularly effective at encouraging these in their adherents.

Finally, in addition to the pleasurable life (SWB) and the meaningful life (PWB), the third psychological dimension of wellbeing is the engaged life (Peterson et al., 2005). The idea of engaged wellbeing (EWB) grew out of the studies of Csikszentmihalyi (1990). He found that when people were asked to report on the type of experiences they found most rewarding, they highlighted activities which were *absorbing*, rather than strictly pleasurable or meaningful. These were passions, from piano playing to rock climbing, that people became engrossed in. Csikszentmihalyi labelled the psychological state produced by these activities as 'flow', as people reported a sense of 'flowing' with the action: attention is completely focused on the activity, sense of self is lost, and time passes quickly. Flow is produced when one's skills are matched to the task at hand, with the activity neither too demanding as to be stressful, nor too easy as to be boring. EWB is different from SWB and PWB as it is 'non-emotional and arguably non-conscious' (Peterson et al., 2005, p. 27). That is, while positive emotions are experienced in retrospect (after engagement), they are not experienced at the time, as one is 'not present'.

From a psychological perspective, SWB, PWB and EWB together comprise the different dimensions of wellbeing as articulated by positive psychology. However, it is recognised that these dimensions – particularly SWB – are also affected by social factors, or what we might call 'contextual determinants' of wellbeing. Finally, it is these factors we consider next.

Social dimensions of wellbeing

In considering the social dimensions of wellbeing, researchers usually examine which aspects of our circumstances impact upon life satisfaction; i.e., using SWB as the dependent variable. Before looking at some of the key factors, it is worth briefly considering a theoretical model to account for why social factors are important, namely a telic – i.e., goal satisfaction – theory of wellbeing. Such theories present individuals as existing in a transactional relationship with the environment; wellbeing is the result of the environment satisfying basic biopsychological needs (Diener et al., 1999). There are various theories of needs. For example, Doyle and Gough (1991) outline 11 universal needs, the deprivation of which detrimentally impacts upon wellbeing, including nutrition, healthcare and relationships. Some theories are hierarchical, most famously Maslow's (1943) model, where as basic physiological needs are met, more abstract ones assume importance, like self-esteem. In contrast, others argue that there are trade-offs between different needs – that supportive relationships can minimise the impact of material deprivation, for example (Biswas-Diener & Diener, 1991).

We can now consider the four most important social factors for wellbeing, as identified by the World Values Survey (Helliwell & Putnam, 2004). The most important factor is close, loving relationships, and marriage in particular (more than cohabitation, as married couples are less likely to part) (Nakhaie & Arnold, 2010). A survey of 59,000 people in 42 countries found a consistent relationship between wellbeing and marital status (Diener et al., 2000). Conversely, the greatest depressant of wellbeing is separation, followed by widowhood (Blanchflower & Oswald, 2004). Although there are some selection effects before the age of 30 – happier people are more likely to marry – this does not apply to those getting married over 30, for whom the positive relationship with wellbeing still holds (Stutzer & Frey, 2006). One theory for the positive impact of marriage is that it offers various 'protection' effects which enhance wellbeing, including division of labour, companionship, and emotional support from people sharing similar goals and ideals (levels of wellbeing are higher in marriages involving similar personalities) (Arrindell & Luteijn, 2000).

The second most important factor is one's financial situation. Socio-economic factors are an important determinant of mental health. For example, men in the lowest socio-economic class in England are almost three times more likely to have CMDs than men in the highest (EHRC, 2011). Such effects are found cross-culturally (Lund et al., 2010). There are environmental factors associated with poverty, like reduced social capital (e.g., community trust; see below) in deprived areas, reflected in higher rates of social disorder (Ross, 2000). Income per se also affects wellbeing, though the correlation is relatively weak (around 0.2; Lucas & Schimmack, 2009). However, this association is mediated by wealth: rises in income increase wellbeing for poorer people (allowing basic needs to be met), but the impact diminishes as wealth rises (Ferrer-i-Carbonell, 2005). As such, despite rising prosperity over the last quarter of the 20th century in Britain, wellbeing has stagnated (Blanchflower & Oswald, 2004). An explanation here is that wellbeing is more affected by relative income (social comparison) than absolute income. As general prosperity rises, this just raises the bar in terms of what is deemed success (Easterlin, 1995). Moreover, inequality in Western societies means people make invidious comparisons with the better off, lowering their wellbeing (Hagerty, 2000).

The third factor is work. Wellbeing can be adversely affected by both being in work and out of work. In work, various factors can serve to decrease wellbeing, from demanding work with little personal control (as per the job demand–control theory; Karasek, 1997) to a mismatch between efforts and rewards (as per the effort–reward imbalance theory; Siegrist, 1996). Wellbeing is also diminished by job insecurity, an issue of increasing relevance, reported by 1 in 5 of the UK workforce (Meltzer et al., 2010). Out of work, even after adjusting for the effects of loss of income, unemployment reduces wellbeing, and leads to increases in CMDs (Pittau et al., 2010). Moreover, long-term unemployment is an exception to the hedonic treadmill – people rarely adapt (Lucas et al., 2004). The impact of unemployment may be lessened where it is a social 'norm', i.e., areas of high unemployment, where other people are similarly suffering (Clark et al., 2010). However, Pittau et al. (2010) argue that this is not the case: no matter how others fare, being out of work still drags down happiness.

Finally, friends and community are the fourth factor. Good social networks impact positively on wellbeing, and protect against stress (Helliwell & Putnam, 2004). This effect is direct: one can turn to others for support. It is also indirect: community cohesion has a positive impact on other factors which also affect wellbeing – known as 'externalities' – such as crime levels. A useful theoretical notion here is Bourdieu's (1986, p. 248) concept of social capital, i.e., the 'sum total of the resources, actual or virtual, that accrue to an individual (or a group) by virtue of being enmeshed in a durable network of more or less institutionalized relationships of mutual acquaintance and recognition'. Social capital is a subtle concept, with a number of different aspects. Bonding is the connectedness within social groups, while bridging refers to good relations between different groups. It can be seen as both a cognitive attribute (attitudes such as trust in people), and a structural phenomenon (network connections, like membership in voluntary organisations). It can also be considered on a micro level (resources available to people to call upon), and a macro level (a community-level resource, enabling achievement of goals that people could not manage alone). A large body of work has consistently shown that social capital is a vital aspect of wellbeing (Jorgensen et al., 2010).

So, we can see that wellbeing comprises multiple dimensions, each of which are themselves multifaceted. Physical wellbeing involves (relative) freedom from illness and disease, as well as efforts people make to promote their health, such as taking exercise. With psychological wellbeing, from a 'negative' perspective, this means (relative) freedom from distress and mental health disorders. We have also seen that stressful life events can contribute to distress, although the impact of these can be mitigated by the skilful use of adaptive coping strategies, and good emotional management generally. From a 'positive' perspective, we have looked at three different 'types' of wellbeing. Subjective wellbeing refers to hedonic pleasure and satisfaction with life. Psychological wellbeing involves meaning in life, psychological growth, self-determination and intrinsic goals. Engaged wellbeing results from absorbing activities. Finally, we have seen that contextual social factors can contribute to wellbeing, notably close relationships, a certain level of financial security, employment and a good social network. All of these dimensions will be relevant throughout this book, as we trace the way in which the men interviewed here tried to engage with wellbeing in all its different aspects. Before commencing our journey with these men however, I shall say a little about who they are, and how they came to share their stories with me.

The interviews

In order to explore the relationship between masculinity and wellbeing, I wanted to interview men about their experiences relating to wellbeing. In particular, I wanted to talk to men who had found ways to engage positively with their wellbeing. In this way, I could challenge the idea – often encountered in academic literature and in society at large – that men are universally poor at taking care of themselves, and that masculinity inevitably has a detrimental impact on wellbeing. I decided to focus on men who meditate. The reason for this decision will become clear in the course of this book. Suffice to say that there is considerable interest in academic and clinical circles around the potential for meditation to improve wellbeing (Brown et al., 2007). For example, reviews assessing the evidence from multiple studies have concluded that practising meditation can help reduce levels of depression and anxiety, and promote SWB (Mars & Abbey, 2010).

Firstly, I needed to find meditators to talk to. To start with, I attended meditation centres and events attended by meditators in London. At these, I first spoke with 'gatekeepers' – people who can provide access to other people and resources – such as the leaders of the meditation centres, to get their approval and/or help with recruitment. I then put up posters, handed out flyers, and generally mentioned that I was undertaking research on meditation to anyone I met. Gradually, men began to volunteer for interviews. Many of these came from a particular meditation centre that I was attending personally on a regular basis. As promised to those I interviewed, to preserve the anonymity of this centre, I will not name it. Nor will I include the real names of the participants, or details that might identify them.

When selecting men to interview, I aimed for an ideal of maximum variation sampling. This meant looking for a wide range of demographic backgrounds and life experience among the participants. I believe I managed to do this. In all, 30 men were recruited. They varied in age from 27 to 61. A few left formal schooling at 16, many had university degrees, and some had professional qualifications. Occupations ranged from transport workers to teachers, graphic designers to doctors. Most men were white – possibly reflecting a general trend in 'converts' to meditation in Britain (Smith, 2008) – with only a few from ethnic minority backgrounds. Nine of the men identified as homosexual, and 21 as heterosexual. Some were single, many had partners, and quite a few had families. Finally, their meditation history ranged from 27 years of experience, to one man who had taken it up just a few months previously. Some practised for as little as 20 minutes each week, others over an hour every day.

The interviews lasted around two hours. The aim was to elicit men's narratives of meditation. This meant asking them to tell their life story, explaining how they came to start meditation, and the effect it had had on their lives and their wellbeing. I did not have set questions. Instead, I had an opening invitation designed to prompt a narrative: 'Can you tell me a bit about life before meditation?' This was chosen as sufficiently open-ended to allow men to begin their story at the point and in the way they felt to be most important, and encouraged the inclusion of any aspects of life they felt to be relevant. Most started talking about their childhood, then traced their story up to the present. Interjections were used to draw out the narratives (e.g., 'Then what happened?'). After men had finished their story, topics of interest were followed up. This meant returning to episodes in the story that warranted revisiting for more detail, and inquiring about topics (if not already covered) around wellbeing. The aim was always to steer the discussion away from abstract reflections, and on to specific experiences in men's lives. In addition, a year later, I conducted a follow-up interview, which lasted about an hour; the process was the same as for the first, except here I sought narratives of the intervening year (which I elicited by asking: 'Can you tell me a bit about this year?').

I chose to explore narratives as they are a means of 'understanding experience as lived and told' (Savin-Baden & Niekerk, 2007, p. 459). That is, narratives reflect both experience itself and the way a person represents this to themselves and others. This distinction broadly reflects Ricoeur's (1981) differentiation between a hermeneutics of 'faith' and of 'suspicion'.

The former involves an 'empathic-interpretative' perspective in which we 'trust' the teller's account about their experiences. The latter recognises the performative functions of narrative as people construct self-identities through discourse. Together, the two perspectives provide a 'more complete understanding of the participant's lived experience' (Frost et al., 2010, p. 15).

Similarly, Xu and Connelly (2009) distinguish between narrative-as-method and narrative-as-phenomenon. As method, they offer information about past experiences, and thus overlap with approaches like life-history research. Such approaches have been criticised over the historical veracity of the data, with issues around memory, and people's tendency to construct stories that uphold positive self-interpretations (Duff & Bell, 2002). Yet from a perspective of narrative-as-phenomenon, regardless of historical accuracy, narratives are an overarching code for the way people construct, understand, and transmit meanings about their identity, past and life (White, 1987). As Frank (1997, p. 22) says, 'The stories we tell about our lives are not necessarily those lives as they were lived, but those stories become our experience of those lives.' Thus, without denying the potential for narratives to reflect lived experience – as this would do injustice to people's efforts to truthfully share their lives (Connell, 1995) – narratives reveal how people think about their life, which itself is important for wellbeing.

Finally, I should say a little about how the narratives were analysed. I used a form of analysis called 'modified constant comparison' (MCC), a derivation of a method known as 'modified grounded theory' (MGT) (Strauss & Corbin, 1998). Both MCC and MGT identify emergent themes through a bottom-up, data-driven inductive process. MCC follows most of the steps of MGT, but falls short of the final step of developing a theoretical framework. Instead, there is a more modest aim of trying to articulate the interrelationships between the key themes, and produce explanations. The prefix 'modified' is appended to indicate that one may turn to existing concepts in the literature to help develop and clarify the emergent themes. (This contrasts with the intent of the originators of grounded theory, Glaser and Strauss (1967), who said that the emergent analysis should be 'purely' grounded in the data.) Thus, while the data was in the form of narratives, MCC was used to look for common themes that would enable the development of explanations that fitted all the interviews (while being guided by relevant evidence/theories in the literature) (Cutcliffe, 2005). The aim was not to make sweeping generalisations, but to explore the relationships between themes 'discovered' in the data. The analysis involved a number of stages. In MCC, data collection (interviews) and analysis happen concurrently, informing each other in a cyclical way, rather than a linear sequence. However, for the sake of clarity, I will briefly describe the analytic process in stages.

The first stage was reading of the transcript(s) to gain an overall impression of the data. The second stage involved 'open-coding'; transcripts were examined thoroughly for themes. This process had two phases. First, in an expansive way, codes were noted exhaustively, with no restriction on the number of codes, which generated over 500, many very narrow. A phase of consolidation was thus necessary, merging codes that were overly specific (e.g., 'happiness' and 'joy' into 'positive emotions'), or subsuming codes into more general ones, reducing the codes to around 100. The next step was organising codes by grouping them under higher headings, according to conceptual similarity. This created a hierarchical tree-structure two levels deep: codes and categories. The next stage was *axial* coding, involving exploration of combinations of codes in order to examine interrelations between them. The final stage was developing a tentative explanatory framework. This involved identifying concepts by taking combinations from the previous stage, and articulating the relationships between them. For example, three significant combinations were 'masculinity and alcohol', 'masculinity and social pressure' and 'coping and distress'. The relationships between these combinations produced two concepts: men drinking to fit in, and men drinking as a coping strategy. These concepts helped form the explanatory framework, which provides the substance of this book.

Having explained how the ideas contained in this book were identified, we can now start to explore the narratives of the men I interviewed. We will follow their journeys, from youth to the present day. These journeys will help illustrate the connections between masculinity and wellbeing. We begin in the next chapter with their tales of childhood and adolescence. This will allow us to explore how boys are subjected to masculinity pressures, which consequently informs the kind of men they become. Through the analysis, we will be able to see common themes among men's experiences of this period of life. Subsequent chapters will then show respectively how men turned to meditation, learned to develop awareness of their inner world through their practice, and then were able to use this awareness to engage constructively with their wellbeing. Throughout the book, I will use actual quotes from participants to illustrate my points, although the men themselves will only be referred to using a pseudonym.

Summary

This chapter introduced two bodies of work that are central to this book, pertaining to gender and wellbeing. With gender, we introduced various conventional approaches, including biological (sex-differences), social (learned roles and stereotypes) and psychological (gender-identity) perspectives. However, we saw how more recent social constructionist theorising emphasises diversity both in men themselves and in masculine norms which shape behaviour. We then looked at wellbeing, which was identified as comprising multiple dimensions, each of which are themselves multifaceted. Physical wellbeing involves (relative) freedom from illness and disease. Psychologically, wellbeing can be defined in a 'negative' way (the relative absence of distress and mental illness) and a positive way (the presence of SWB, PWB, and EWB). Finally, contextual social factors contribute to wellbeing, such as close relationships and a good social network. The rest of the book will explore the fascinating, complex, troubling, and ultimately hopeful intersections between these two bodies of work. These intersections will be illustrated, contextualised, and illuminated in the experiences of the men whose narratives form the substance of this book. I hope you enjoy following their journeys.

2
Becoming a Man

I never saw [my father] cry until he had his breakdown. He was very controlled, he didn't allow the softer side out. I just took that from him, that's how you should be. (Dalton)

We now begin our journey, following the stories of the men I interviewed. Eventually we will find out how meditation practice enhanced their lives and their wellbeing. Before this though, we want to trace the reasons men began meditation, and the struggles they faced in reaching that point. As such, we start at the beginning, looking at their formative years, their accounts of childhood and adolescence. Here we shall see the way my participants were influenced and shaped by cultural expectations around masculinity as they learned to become 'a man'. It will also become clear that these expectations had a detrimental impact on many participants. In particular, we will examine the corrosive impact of norms around toughness and strength, and the way these led men to become disconnected from their emotions. Furthermore, we will see how this emotional disconnection had a deleterious impact upon participants' wellbeing.

Childhood: Learning masculinity

As my participants traced their journeys towards their engagement with meditation, many began their story in childhood. For many, this was depicted as a period of innocence. It is important that I do not give the false impression that all men had similar stories. Although my analysis focused on common themes in the narratives, I was also keen to explore complexity, to find the exceptions to the rule, the deviations from the norm. As such, whenever I make assertions about the experiences of 'many' or 'most' men, there is always the implicit caveat that this assertion by no means applies to all participants. Moreover, I will try to highlight complexities wherever possible, and point out the exceptions. Nevertheless, I will weave this presentation out of common threads, and try to give a sense of the points of convergence in men's stories, highlighting experiences that many men shared. In this sense, it is accurate to say that most men recalled their childhood in quite idyllic terms. Kris (a pseudonym), who was one of the younger men in my sample, recalled a happy childhood abroad. He described spending hours surfing with his mates as part of a small rural beach community:

> *It was like paradise really, it was beautiful ... I've got a huge family ... We had a real group, a little tribe, plus all of our friends.*

As we consider his evocative statement, it is worth pausing for a moment to contemplate the nature of narrative. It is fairly self-evident that all childhoods will contain a broad spectrum of experiences, featuring – unless an extremely unusual and atypical childhood – a mixture of positive and negative events. Thus we would not dare assert that Kris's childhood was free of problems, that his memory contains no dark fragments from that period. No doubt that if we probed his childhood in depth, we would uncover some painful recollections. However, it is also true to say that, overall, he presented a story of a happy childhood. From the perspective of Ricoeur's (1981) hermeneutics of faith, this points to a truth about his actual childhood – it was experienced *at the time* as generally happy. From the perspective of a hermeneutics of suspicion, the narrative is more reflective of how Kris portrays his childhood to himself *in the present*, which need not necessarily bear resemblance to the way it actually occurred. Some scholars argue that we need to pick one of these perspectives (faith or suspicion). However, Ricoeur urged people to keep both perspectives in mind, that narratives can tell us something genuine about the past (faith), but are subject to revision in the present (suspicion). Thus, as a general principle here, we will adopt a similarly balanced hermeneutics of faith and suspicion to all the narratives in the book.

As such, we can trust Kris that his childhood was generally as he depicted it, i.e., happy, safe and connected. Yet we can also grant that he is using some poetic licence in how he portrays it. Indeed, the notion that childhood is (or should be) an idyllic period of safety is a powerful romantic discourse in Western society (Horton, 2008). This depiction of childhood essentially draws its power from the way it is vividly contrasted with the relative harshness of adulthood. With many men, the image of a blissful childhood did seem to have been evoked precisely to emphasise how difficult it was transitioning to adulthood. To adapt a biblical metaphor, many men portrayed childhood as a lost Eden, before a loss of innocence and the fall into adulthood. A number of men described childhood as a bubble, protecting them from the sharper edges of the world. However, within these stories, the function of this Edenic image was to presage a painful descent, a troubled awakening to the difficulties of existence. Some men mourned the loss of this protective bubble, of a time when life was uncomplicated: *'There was a church up the road, and the primary school ... a safe, protected bubble ... We were all very, very happy'* (William). For some men though, there was even an accusatory note in their voice when they lamented being unprepared for what was to come.

> *I don't think my peaceful, quiet upbringing really prepared me for the harsh realities of life ... I was always able to turn away. [Then later], when they hit you in the face, you're just not able to cope with them.* (Dean)

Before we discuss this 'fall' into adulthood, it is important to emphasise – as I will seek to do throughout this book – that not all stories were the same. In contrast to the Edenic narratives above, a few men depicted their childhood in wholly damning terms. These men portrayed no time of safety before the fall; the world was recalled as unforgiving from the start. Indeed, it is suggested that recollections of childhood tend to cleave to extremes, painted in floral terms as either a heaven or a hell (Neustadter, 2004). For example, Robert described his early years as *'hostile, bad, conflict-zone, war-zone, difficulties, bullying, beatings up, abuse'*. A similar tale of hardship was told by Michael, who recalled bullying at the hands of his older brothers. What makes Michael's story so relevant to the central message of this chapter is that his difficulties foreshadow the kinds of issues that would soon trouble most participants: he was bullied because he did not live up to expectations about how boys should be. Michael, who is gay, portrayed himself as an effeminate child. Consequently, he was subject to *'constant taunting'* from his *'traditionally masculine'* older brothers. Thus, here we find the first mention of the idea that boys growing up face social pressures to act in certain ways. In particular, behaviours viewed as stereotypically feminine are 'policed' by forms of societal 'censure', i.e., discouraged through social penalties of varying severity (Roberts, 1993).

> *I wasn't like the strapping lads that my brothers are ... I used to cry very easily and so they'd like to make me cry ... They taunted me for weakness*

and effeteness...I didn't fit in to the world I was brought up in...My parents [said], 'You must stand up to them', [but I] was never very good at that and never did. I was very, very unhappy.

Michael and Robert had a relatively early introduction to life's troubles. As such, they also gained an early sense that they might need to be tough to deal with this. More crucially, they also become aware that they were *expected* to be tough. For the majority of other participants, who depicted a carefree childhood, such realisations came slightly later, in early adolescence.

More specifically, a number of participants located 13 as the age at which childhood ended – the threshold into adulthood. Descriptions of this threshold were often linked to certain events which burst the *'bubble'* of childhood, awakening the boys to a harsher existence. Colin had a *'wakeup'* as his mother's drinking problem *'descended into oblivion'* and she became *'violent and neglectful'*. At this point, his *'really happy childhood came down from fantasy to reality'*. Steven's dad left the family *'with very little notice'* to live with a new partner. The family had to move *'to a cramped little house the other side of the town'*, and Steven *'stepped into a head of the family sort of role'*. Ernest was *'badly beaten up'* by an older family member; he immediately left home and *'spent the next ten years being passed from pillar to post'*. For a number of boys, the threshold occurred when they switched from a smaller primary school – where they had felt comfortable and safe – to a larger, more challenging secondary school.

I had a very happy, stable family upbringing in suburbia, a safe, protected bubble. The big change happened when I went to secondary school. That was my first experience of life as a tough, hard environment. (William)

It is at this point – the threshold – that themes of toughness really come to the fore in men's narratives. There were two aspects to this. Some boys tried to be physically and emotionally tough as a way of coping, of protecting themselves. For example, growing up in a rough part of London, Alvin described his *'teenage aggression'* as a *'survival strategy'*. Indeed, at-risk youth are often more in danger of adopting antisocial (i.e., aggressive) coping strategies than boys with more affluent upbringings (Blechman & Culhane, 1993). However, others did not necessarily *want* to be tough, but were told by those around them that *as boys* they should be, just as Michael experienced earlier on. Thus here we see the inculcation of gendered norms, as depicted by social learning theorists. As Morrongiello and Dawber (2000) found, by buying into conventional gender stereotypes, parents have a strong influence on boys' learned behaviour. For example, through his childhood, Dalton's mother had told him stories about his grandfather: *'He was as tough as old boots, he didn't have "emotions".'* These messages were ubiquitous and persuasive: *'There was a lot of that growing up... "You don't want to be soft, you don't want to be wet".'* Like other boys, Dalton had a *'tough time'* switching to secondary school. At this point, his mother's stories about his grandfather really hit home. He gives a vivid account of suddenly crossing the threshold, and needing to be 'a man'.

> *I remember having a sense of, 'I'm grown up now.' It seemed to happen overnight. It was like, 'I shouldn't cry anymore', almost like I just decided that. So I hardly cried. Whereas when I was a child it [crying] came fairly easily, relief, then it would go. When I was about 13, it was like ssswww-pppp. I went to a new school, had quite a difficult time, I thought, 'I've got to face this alone.' It was this myth of being the lone man, the myth from my grandfather...My dad was [also] like that. I never saw him cry until he had his breakdown. He was very controlled, he didn't allow the softer side out. I just took that from him, that's how you should be.*

This is a pivotal excerpt, highlighting themes which are central to this book. It vividly shows how men are encouraged to disconnect from their emotions, as will be discussed at length below. More generally, it shows how boys are socialised into manhood. This has implications for our view of masculinity. Essentialist theories, especially biologically-based approaches to gender, tend to assume that the 'male character' is somewhat 'fixed' from birth on account of male physiology (Eagly & Wood, 1999). On this view, boys are just small men. However, analysing discourse used by 9–13-year-olds, Mac an Ghaill and Haywood (2012) found that boys' identities fluctuated between an adult masculinity and a 'feminised' childhood. This reflects Dalton's narrative, in which qualities perceived as 'feminine' – such as crying – were permitted in childhood but were increasingly discouraged as he crossed the threshold. On this evidence, then, it is not that males are unemotional, but they learn to be as they are taught to 'be a man'. Thus, although children are aware of conventions around gender from a young age (even as early as 18 months; Eichstedt et al., 2002), it is in adolescence when gender becomes a really 'salient factor shaping orientations toward oneself and views of one's place in the social world' (Barrett & White, 2002, p. 451).

This pressure to be tough came not only from parents. Other key sources included peers, and the media. In participants' accounts of adolescence, 'fitting in' with peers was a prominent concern. Previous work has shown that adolescent boys are under considerable pressure to enact traditional hegemonic forms of masculinity – such as being tough, cool or sporty – to avoid the censure and bullying that comes with being seen as 'feminine' (Frosh et al., 2003). Youths who challenge traditional hegemonic expectations face considerable mistreatment at school from their peers. For example, homosexuality is generally seen as a marginalised form of masculinity, subject to societal censure: 83 per cent of LGBT people in the UK report having experienced discrimination or hostility related to their sexuality (Warner et al., 2004). At school, over half of LGBT pupils report experiencing homophobic bullying, and 99 per cent have encountered homophobic discourses (Guasp, 2012). This bullying is related to an increased risk of suicidal ideation and behaviour, with LGBT boys between 2 and 12 times more likely to attempt suicide than heterosexual boys (Saewyc et al., 2008). Moreover, schools as institutions can be complicit in this homophobic censure: 3 in 5 LGBT pupils say that teachers who witness homophobic acts do not intervene (Guasp, 2012). This systemic complicity of schools in homophobia, and in inculcating traditional gender norms generally, has been labelled 'poisonous pedagogy' (Kenway & Fitzclarence, 1997).

Consequently, most participants reported pressure to fit in and avoid bullying, including gay participants, many of whom were compelled to hide their sexuality (discussed further below). Unfortunately, the type of behaviours that boys felt they needed to enact to be accepted by peers usually followed traditional masculine norms around aggression and risk-taking. These types of low-level antisocial behaviours have been given the label 'laddishness', including ' "having a laugh", alcohol consumption, disruptive behaviour', etc. (Francis, 1999, p. 357). In light of the bullying faced by boys who do not conform to the traditional expectations, rather than laddishness being a natural propensity – 'boys will be boys' – it could be seen as a self-protection strategy, driven by fear of being stigmatised as feminine (Jackson, 2002). Mejía (2005) refers to this socially-learned toughness as a 'shame-hardening process', inculcating the potent message that 'boys don't cry'. Thus acting tough may be driven by vulnerability, a fear of being different. Moreover, adopting a 'cool pose' of 'bravado' may also be a way of *concealing* vulnerability, erecting an 'impenetrable wall of toughness' to protect oneself (Pollack, 2006, p. 191). These ideas were demonstrated vividly by Ernest. He tried to emulate the aggressive iconography of hip-hop – showing the power of masculine imagery conveyed in the media in shaping boys' constructions of self-identity (Dimitriadis, 2009) – to conceal his vulnerabilities.

> *I was trying to emulate some kind of manhood, seeking symbols of macho-ism, sexual conquests, being anarchic, not conforming. A lot of that came from feeling insecure. [Rappers] have a swagger, an attitude, they carry a confidence. To not feel anxiety, that's what it stems from.*

It is important at this juncture to once again highlight differences within men's stories. It was striking that nearly all participants reported coming up against pressure to enact traditional forms of hegemonic masculinity, e.g., being tough. However, not all participants succumbed to this pressure. Whether they did or not seemed to depend largely on the type of upbringing they experienced as they crossed the 'threshold'. Across all the narratives, three main types of family relationships during the threshold period were described. These had certain parallels with Bowlby's (1973) theory of attachment. Attachment theory concerns the relative security of early interpersonal relationships, particularly the mother–infant bond, and the effect these have on subsequent development. As developed by various scholars, notably Ainsworth et al. (1979), the theory differentiates between secure attachment and two types of insecure attachment, avoidant and ambivalent. A secure attachment gives the child the confidence to explore the world, safe in the knowledge that their attachment figure will not disappear. With insecure attachments, this confidence is lacking: infants with ambivalent bonds become very distressed if separated from a caregiver, while those with avoidant bonds are emotionally passive and detached. Although Bowlby's theory concerns early childhood, while participants here were discussing adolescence, the theory is still relevant, since attachment styles formed in infancy often persist in later life (Ravitz et al., 2010).

However, in contrast to standard attachment theory, narratives here featured one main type of insecure attachment, and *two* types of secure attachment. The insecure attachment took the form of a 'dysfunctional' family situation as participants crossed the threshold, with a relative absence of familial support. Ernest, who acted tough to hide his vulnerability, as noted above, depicted this type of upbringing: '*At 13 I was badly beaten up by [a relative]. I left home, spent the next ten years being passed from pillar to post, not having a sense of place...all the while trying to develop a sense of my own identity and manhood...[I] ended up getting involved in gangs, smoking a lot of weed.*' In contrast were two types of secure attachment. The first of these could be called 'facilitative', involving a caring, nurturing environment that encouraged independence, as described by Sam: '*[My parents] found it important I live my life the way I wanted. They were concerned...but always very supportive...I could shape my life in my own way.*' A second type of secure attachment might be described as 'over-secure'. This 'constrictive' attachment consisted of a caring yet overbearing bond which discouraged independence, recalled by John as '*smothering*': '*Went to university, got a job...Not much awareness of anything else...Always family pressures. I didn't realise I had a choice.*'

The importance of these different familial circumstances during the threshold period was that they seemed to impact on participants' ability to resist traditional hegemonic norms. The few who reported being better able to resist hegemonic pressures connected this to a 'facilitative' upbringing. For example, with homosexuality censured as noted above, most gay participants recalled considerable difficulties accepting their sexuality (see below). However, with a supportive family who encouraged his independence, Sam had '*no problem with it*', and came out in his mid-teens. In contrast, boys with dysfunctional or constrictive upbringings had greater difficulties resisting traditional expectations, but for quite different reasons. For those with dysfunctional families, lack of familial support as the boys crossed the threshold accentuated their sense of vulnerability. This vulnerability encouraged toughness – emotional and physical – as a way of coping. For example, as Ernest described above, lacking parental support he sought security in teenage gangs and the aggression of hip-hop. Conversely, for boys with 'constrictive' bonds, although they felt cared for, their independence was not nurtured. Consequently, they were less able to challenge hegemonic expectations. For example, Ali later fulfilled his ambition to work as a nurse. However, for many years he had been unable to pursue this career, since he did not want to go against his parents, who saw it as '*something a girl does*'.

As Ali's story indicates, it was not necessarily the case that participants from constrictive or dysfunctional upbringings *wanted* to conform to traditional masculine expectations, but more that they lacked the support to do so. This was not true of all those from such backgrounds – as John intimated above, he did not have '*much awareness*' of other options available to him. However, others from constrictive backgrounds wanted to challenge the restrictions placed on them. Ross recalled an '*impulse to break out and find something bigger*', escaping the narrow confines of the traditional gender roles seemingly open to him. It was possible for men to resist such pressures and break free from convention, as those with a facilitative background were encouraged to do. However, for boys with restrictive upbringings, doing so risked facing disapproval from families, or worse.

For example, Harry wanted to pursue an artistic career that his very traditional working-class father regarded as unmasculine, and *'couldn't tell his mates'* about. Harry was determined to follow his ambitions, and told a tragic story of being disowned by his parents (*'How I really coped, I don't know. I turned my back on them'*). Unfortunately, it is not uncommon for children who challenge conventional gender norms – such as boys who are gay – to face disapproval, shame and even rejection from their families (LaSala, 2000). This can add to the pressure to conform to hegemonic expectations.

The impact of upbringing on boys' susceptibility to traditional hegemonic norms introduces another interesting dimension to the narratives: the importance of taking 'intersectionality' into account. Intersectionality refers to the way different identity categories impact upon each other to create complexities within each particular category (Hankivsky & Christoffersen, 2008). This perspective highlights the limitations of treating any one identity category, such as gender, in isolation. For example, socio-economic status (SES) intersects with masculinity to produce differences in mental health: men in the poorest fifth of the population are almost three times more likely to suffer a common mental disorder than men in the richest fifth (EHRC, 2011). In the narratives here, the family situations that were reported as being dysfunctional or constrictive were usually, though not always, families that were of lower SES. In contrast, families where there was a facilitative bond appeared more likely to have higher SES. For example, Sam – who I have presented as an exemplar of a facilitative upbringing – described an affluent childhood as *'the fifth child of a fairly rich family ... We weren't spoilt, but there was plenty of money.'* In contrast, Alvin recalled an upbringing that was poor and relatively dysfunctional. His narrative of youth was full of stories about enacting traditional hegemonic norms, such as aggression.

> *I was the child of a single parented family, my mum had me when she was 17, I left home at 15, had a child at 18, started working at 13, you see, and it kind of shapes you, as a person ... In hindsight, perhaps that aggression was something that I needed, it was a survival instinct.*

This contrast between Alvin and Sam – between dysfunctional and facilitative upbringings – reflects work by Jones (2002), who analysed transitions into adulthood. Jones suggested that there were different 'paths' taken by youths: a 'slow track' and a 'fast track'. The former describes a process of crossing and re-crossing boundaries between childhood and adulthood in a series of partial transitions between dependence and independence. This 'track' relies on parental support until the youth acquires social/cultural capital, mainly through educational attainments. Clearly, this track has parallels with the 'facilitative' upbringing identified here. In contrast, as the name implies, the fast track involves a sudden transition, characterised by negative physical and emotional experiences as the youth is thrust – somewhat unprepared – into adulthood. This track reflects the path taken by participants in my research who recalled dysfunctional upbringings. Moreover, as with my findings, Jones argued that SES influences the track taken, with disadvantaged youths more likely to take the fast track. Alvin continued his narrative by emphasising how his dysfunctional family situation had forced him sharply over the threshold – much as Steven suggested that he had to '*suddenly*' take over '*a head of the family sort of role*' at 13 when his father left – propelling him on a fast track to adulthood.

> *As a very young boy, I would be like 11, 12, on my own, looking after my sister, my mum would be at work until 8 o'clock at night.*

Furthermore, as I also found, Jones reported that fast-track youths are more likely to engage in traditional destructive masculine behaviours, like aggression. I have suggested that such behaviours may be a coping strategy, a way of dealing with a rough social situation. It has also been argued that men with less power in society – like those with lower SES – are often compelled to compensate by demonstrating 'hypermasculine' behaviours, such as violence (although we shall take issue below with this term 'hypermasculine'). That is, hegemonic masculinity is intrinsically bound up with issues of power, with assertion of power a marker of successful attainment of hegemonic status; i.e., powerful men have successfully proved themselves to be 'real' men. Men with powerful jobs or wealth can draw on their high social standing as a way of demonstrating power (Connell & Wood, 2005). This option is foreclosed to men with less standing, who may resort to cruder means of assertion, such as aggression (Lutze & Bell, 2005). Back in 1927, the psychoanalyst Adler described such compensatory attempts to assert one's manhood as the 'masculine protest' (Adler, 1927). Moreover, Adler highlighted the way such performances were driven by insecurity, and fear of being perceived as feminine. Such ideas were echoed by Ernest, who depicted his quest to emulate the '*machoism*' of hip-hop as an act.

Around 17, 18, 19, I was starting to become aware that although that attitude, that urban swagger, that hip hop lifestyle and the trouble I got into was appealing... it was a façade.

Young adulthood: The emotional consequences of masculinity

So far, this chapter has suggested that many boys growing up were influenced by traditional masculine norms, such as emotional toughness. Whether out of a concern with fitting in and avoiding being censured for seeming feminine, or as a coping strategy for dealing with one's vulnerabilities, many participants worked hard to live up to these norms. This however had serious consequences for their wellbeing. From mid-adolescence onwards, many participants experienced significant psychological and social difficulties as a result of their attempts to be tough. There were four main issues: boys became *disconnected from others*; some young men felt a creeping sense of *inauthenticity* (as revealed by Ernest, when he spoke about his *'urban swagger'* being a *'façade'*); participants took on the message that aspects of their person (e.g., feelings of sadness) were unacceptable, and as a result experienced *inner conflict*; finally, from trying to be emotionally tough, participants became *disconnected from their inner world*, with deleterious consequences. This section looks at these issues in turn.

Disconnection from others

The first consequence of participants' attempts to emulate the traditional masculine norms of toughness and independence was a sense of disconnection from those around. Following the poetic nomenclature used by Dalton above, we might call this the 'lone man' stance. At this point, I want to introduce a pair of concepts that will be helpful in discussing these issues. It is often asserted that men prefer independence, and women prefer building relationships. This assertion is so common that these are frequently viewed as 'masculine' and 'feminine' traits respectively. However, a more useful way of thinking about these two approaches to social life – independence versus connection – is in terms of agency and communion. These notions were developed by Bakan (1966) to reflect the two fundamental dimensions of existence. On one hand, people exist as separate individuals. In this sense, agency refers to the process by which people differentiate themselves from others and develop autonomy as free individuals. On the other hand, apart from in extreme circumstances, people are also part of wider social networks. Communion then refers to the way we build and sustain connections with wider networks that sustain our being, whether physically, emotionally or mentally.

The key point about these two modes of being is that even though they appear diametrically opposed, there is an onus on people to cultivate *both* simultaneously. People are required to develop as autonomous individuals *and* connect with those around. However, navigating this balancing act can be difficult. The philosopher Ken Wilber (1995) has suggested that people can sometimes over-prioritise one of the modes of being, and neglect the other, with adverse consequences. Failure to develop one's autonomy as an individual, instead being subsumed within a larger communion – which Wilber terms 'hypercommunion'– brings the risk of a herd mentality, of being swept along by the crowd. This can have dangerous consequences as people abdicate their self-responsibility and allow their actions to be swayed by group-think. In extreme cases, this can lead to situations such as mob violence, or the mass suicides of religious cults. In contrast, the failure to develop connections with others, instead rigidly pursing one's autonomy – which Wilber calls 'hyperagency' – brings the danger of alienation and isolation.

Wilber suggests that men have a tendency towards hyperagency, which was indeed reflected in the narratives, as discussed below. Before considering examples of such hyperagency, it is worth reflecting on the usefulness of the word. In particular, it avoids fatalistically conflating the qualities it refers to with a particular gender. As noted above, behaviours seen as features of hyperagency – like social disconnectedness or aggression – are sometimes referred to as 'hypermasculine' (Mosher & Tomkins, 1988). The problem with this formulation is that it equates masculinity with a toxic assemblage of traits, and just suggests that some men exhibit these more than others. This overlooks the manifold forms masculinity can take, which is a key message of this book. Taking the example of aggression, not all men are aggressive, and not all forms of masculinity idealise it. Conversely, some females are aggressive, and some forms of femininity valorise it, as with the 'mean girls' archetype (Ringrose, 2006). Thus it is helpful to 'decouple' aggression from any particular gender (while still recognising that men are much more liable to aggression; Ministry of Justice, 2012). This argument applies to all qualities seen as typically masculine or feminine. I recognise that in our society, masculinity is traditionally associated with qualities like toughness; thus, I still use the term 'traditional' masculinity to refer to expectations on men to enact these qualities. However, we will forge a more constructive vision of masculinity if we stop labelling such qualities simplistically as 'masculine'.

So, as reflected in the 'lone man' motif introduced above, participants did indeed describe forms of hyperagency. (Interestingly though, certain aspects of their story were more redolent of hypercommunion, like concern with fitting in – this is discussed further below in relation to inauthenticity.) Many felt they had been disconnected or alienated earlier in life, and some still struggled to shake off that feeling. For example, Richard said: *'I've always felt a bit on my own, a bit out on the outside, not quite connected.'* It was not necessarily that men lacked friends, but that these friendships were often viewed in retrospect as relatively superficial. Jack: *'I had friends but I never had depth … I didn't even know I needed that, never mind how to go about getting it.'* Likewise, Andrew *'knew how to socialise, but I didn't know how to communicate, to really connect with people'*. Reinforcing the notion that toughness can be a way of coping with vulnerability, some described social disconnection as a self-protection strategy. Jack: *'I [didn't] want people to get too close to me because there's probably a fear of getting hurt or something like that.'* Steven suggested he became withdrawn after being thrust over the threshold when his father left home, as detailed above, concealing his parents' separation from his friends. However, he felt his real disconnection from others, especially his family, occurred when his father suddenly returned and he was *'shoved sideways'*.

> *At that point I really cut off from them … just no emotional connection. We were like five separate people by then. And so I can hardly remember leaving home really, it just doesn't mean anything … That actually had great, great repercussions for years … I just wouldn't trust anybody, wouldn't let anybody get close. I had surface friends, but very shallow conversation, nothing deep at all.*

The key point is that men's wellbeing suffered as a result of their disconnection from others. For example, Steven recalled pent-up feelings of shame connected to many issues – like his family background, his later depression – but had been unable to talk to anyone about it (*'Not even my best friend'*). He contrasted this isolation with the community and friendship he had found through meeting other meditators, as explored in later chapters. He now felt the relief of being able to talk to others about his problems, and have their support, and had started to feel his shame *'drifting away'*. Until recently though, he had suffered in his isolation. Men's stories here echo ideas in the literature, which hold that masculine norms around agency, i.e., independence and self-sufficiency, mean that men are generally found to have smaller social networks and fewer close friendships than women (Davidson, 2004). As elucidated in Chapter 1, this has important implications for wellbeing. Close social relationships are one of the key factors in SWB (Helliwell & Putnam, 2004) and PWB (Ryan & Deci, 2000). Social support is also a key resource in coping with physical and mental health problems (Ganster & Victor, 1988). As such, men's generally smaller social networks adversely affect their coping ability (Shiner et al., 2009). Robert suggested that his isolation, which he attributed to him being creatively gifted but socially awkward, led to mental health issues.

> *I had a peer group but I didn't belong to it, not at school nor any-where...People that are gifted, they don't know how to mix in, very often they're very, very imbalanced...I was depressed.*

As ever, it is important to highlight complexity and nuance within the narratives. Not all men felt disconnected; a minority depicted a world of close friendships in their early adulthood. Thus we have a continuum, from isolation to connectedness, with men at various points along this, though skewed more towards the former. As important as acknowledging this variation in men is attempting to understand *why*. Returning to the attachment categorisation, it seemed the few young men who were connected were from facilitative backgrounds. The supportive bonds these men enjoyed gave them strength and wherewithal to resist traditional hegemonic norms, like the 'lone man' ideal. As we shall see, these men were exceptions to many of the negative themes connected to masculinity in this section. Moreover, in the next chapter we shall see that these men were also among the first to find meditation. I have used Sam as my exemplar for someone from a facilitative background. He said his parents *'found it important I live my life the way I wanted'*. He also *'felt different'* because he was gay, yet had plenty of close friends. Through discussions around vegetarianism in his teenage years, his *'conscience was awoken'*. As a result, in his early twenties, he decided – encouraged by his parents – to move into a vegetarian community with other young people who shared his ideals.

> *I liked people and human relationships...I really liked living in a community. There was three guys and three girls...we shared this principle of*

being vegetarian and we had food together and there was a piano in the house, some music after dinner. That was a really good time.

Inauthenticity

Returning now to the travails of the majority of participants who suffered in early adulthood as a result of enacting traditional hegemonic norms, the second issue was inauthenticity. In trying to fit in and live up to traditional masculine ideals, men recalled the pressure to be *'one of the lads'*. At school, this involved being disruptive, and not being studious. In adulthood, it took on darker overtones. For example, Steven depicted his work environment as *'very male, heavy drinking, sexist, racist'*. Thus, despite the 'hyperagentic' pattern of behaviours above, young men were also susceptible to the dangers of hypercommunion. (This highlights the fallacy of identifying agency and communion with masculinity and femininity respectively.) Rather than preserving their autonomy, young men were allowing their values and behaviours to be shaped and even determined by the group. The susceptibility of men to a mob mentality, swept along by a collective fervour into destructive acts, has been analysed in phenomena like football hooliganism (Spaaij, 2008). While participants here did not recall such violent extremes, they did talk about going 'along with the boys'. William attributed his willingness to cede his autonomy to others to a desire to be liked, which was related to low self-esteem.

> *I was always good at being popular, having a laugh, being in the mix ... I just thought the most important thing is to be liked ... I was dependent on everybody topping me up with self-esteem. I thought that by turning myself into what they liked, they would like me. I would go away thinking I was a worthwhile human being.*

However, participants recalled a creeping sense that they were not being 'true' to themselves in some way. Using discourses of 'inauthenticity', they described how trying to attain these traditional masculine expectations began to generate feelings of unease. For some men, these feelings were vague and hard to pin down, just a sense that something wasn't right. As Kris said: *'I was trying to fit in and be one of the lads, when I'm not. Doing things, not being comfortable with it, but not really knowing why.'* For others, their unease was more explicit, being related to the suppression of specific issues. The most vivid narratives in this area relate to sexuality. Nine of the 30 participants were homosexual, and most of these had difficulties coming to terms with this, mainly because it contravened traditional masculine expectations. With the exception of Sam, whose facilitative upbringing meant he had '*no problem*' coming out, all gay participants felt compelled to hide or deny their homosexuality in their youth. These men usually felt unable to come out to peers, and many worried about telling their families. For example, Henry suggested that '*being gay was not an option in my family*'. His sense of inauthenticity and unease came from pretending he wasn't gay, not only concealing this from his parents, but trying to convince himself too.

> *I [wasn't] prepared to share anything with my family, especially when it came to the subject of my sexuality ... It was about pushing it down, pushing it down ... It was denial ... For a long time I had to keep it away from them, I had to keep it away from myself. So I was working really hard at, 'No it's not there.' [I was] in a lot of misery.*

Various schools of thought see the idea of 'authenticity' as central to wellbeing. This includes both existentialism and humanism, which together influenced the contemporary construct of PWB. Existentialist writers make a virtue of authenticity – and allied notions of freedom and autonomy – suggesting people are not living fully if they fail to be authentic (Heidegger, 1927). Similarly, humanist thought has a vision of people as containing innate potentials for growth, each person with particular qualities to develop as they 'become' a unique individual (Rogers, 1961). The notion of authenticity has been criticised, including the accusation that it overlooks the potent constraints of a capitalist economic system that prevents people 'being themselves' (Adorno, 1973). Nevertheless, the concept remains a powerful ideal within many contemporary forms of psychotherapy (Burston & Frie, 2006). Conversely, being *in*authentic also has negative consequences for mental health. Returning to the denial of homosexuality, censure of homosexuality in society may be absorbed by gay people themselves, leading to feelings of self-hatred, referred to as 'internalised homophobia' (Allen & Oleson, 1999). This in turn is linked to mental health issues and suicidality (D'Augelli et al., 2001). Such issues were reported by gay men here, particularly those of the older generation, some of whom grew up when homosexuality was actually illegal.

> *It was an awful time ... Being gay was much more hidden then ... I used to pray that it wasn't true. I remember having nightmares and I used to have these fantasies about having an accident and then being crippled or something, so no-one would ever have to know.* (Michael)

Inner conflict

This poignant quote from Michael leads us into the third main issue connected to masculinity: a sense of inner conflict. Above it was suggested that in conforming to traditional masculine norms, many men felt inauthentic: they were not 'being themselves' around others. We might describe this as a conflict between our public and private selves. The idea that we manage our public personas to conform to situational demands is common. Gough (2001, p. 181) reported that men often withheld non-hegemonic discourses – 'biting their tongue' – around other men out of concern with the 'social costs entailed in appearing "other"'. However, the 'internalised homophobia' that Michael described is altogether more damaging. Here we observe an inner conflict *within* the self, between aspects of the self the person has been encouraged by society to view as acceptable, and aspects they have been coerced into seeing as unacceptable. In Michael's case, these unacceptable aspects were his homosexual feelings. This feeling of an inner split was common among gay participants. They described the painful feeling of being subjected to potent societal messages, including from peers, parents and the media, that their homosexual feelings were wrong. Such pressures contributed to a fractured sense of self; Michael said he came to view the condemned aspects of his character as '*sordid*'.

> *I had to come to terms with this thing ... but I found it very, very difficult ... The worst thing was this awful sense of secrecy and dirtiness. I've grown up with a large portion of guilt [and] almost crippling fear.*

A consequence of this inner conflict is that many gay men tried to deny their homosexuality not only to others but to themselves. Participants described suppressing (curtailing by force) or repressing (holding back) their homosexual feelings. As Henry said: '*It was about pushing it down, pushing it down.*' There is a vast therapeutic literature on repression, not least within psychoanalysis, where Freud (1914) called it 'the cornerstone on which the whole structure' of his theory rested (p. 16). Freud (1915) described repression as 'turning something away, and keeping it at a distance, from the conscious' (p. 147). In this theory, people try to defend themselves against unwanted or undesirable thoughts and feelings by expelling these from consciousness. Crucially however, the repressed material does not disappear, but exercises continual pressure in the direction of the unconscious. The merits of Freud's ideas, and the ways in which repression works, continue to be debated (Billig, 1997). Nevertheless, there is consensus that it is a damaging psychological process. For example, not only does repression take perpetual effort, it actually increases the salience and potency of the repressed material (Wegner & Gold, 1995). Moreover, repression is associated with mental disorders – for example, the continual policing of undesirable thoughts is thought to underpin forms of anxiety, including obsessive compulsive disorder (Ratner & El-Badwi, 2011).

However, whilst I recognise the Freudian roots of the concept of repression, this is not a book about psychoanalysis or Freud's particular theory. Rather, the emphasis is on theories of emotional management. As will become apparent, men's attempts to repress 'unacceptable' aspects of their being had destructive consequences on their ability to constructively deal with their emotions. In particular, attempts to repress unwanted feelings had the catastrophic consequence of discon- necting men from these feelings. For example, with homosexuality still '*a crime*' when Dustin was a teenager, he fought hard to repress his homosexual feelings. As a result, in his twenties, he was '*very repressed [and] emotionally frozen*', and he suggested that he became '*clinically depressed*' as a result. However, it is vital to emphasise that while I have mainly discussed inner conflict and subsequent repression in relation to homosexuality, it was not limited to this – it was just the most vivid example. Most men saw aspects of their self as unacceptable, and tried to repress these. Policed by expectations of traditional masculinity, many grew up to view aspects of the self as 'feminine', and thus to see these as improper. Men echoed Lupton (1998) in claiming that emotionality itself was often feminised, and thus off limits. To recall the excerpt from Dalton cited above:

> *I never saw [my father] cry until he had his breakdown, he was very con-*
> *trolled, he didn't allow the softer side out, he'd never be sad, or upset...I*
> *just took that from him, that's how you should be.*

The key point is that men still felt such feelings, but came to see these as unacceptable. As Dalton continued: '*I thought that there was something wrong with me, having these feelings...I was aware of them bubbling up, this distressed upset feeling, but I thought, "Oh, there's something wrong with me here".*' Here we see a vivid illustration of an idea that is central to this book: men *learn* to become detached from their emotions, rather than being inherently detached simply because they are men. (This is important, as something which is learned can also be *un*learned.) It is commonly suggested that men have tendencies towards 'restric- tive emotionality', i.e., being detached or disconnected from emotions

(Levant, 1992). Sometimes this is referred to using a clinical term – 'alexithymia' – defined as an 'inability to recognize or verbalize emotions' (Honkalampi et al., 2000, p. 99). Such is the prevalence for alexithymia in men that Levant and colleagues (2009) speak of 'normative male alexithymia'. Many participants did indeed describe being emotionally restricted. However, the crucial finding is that this 'affective style' was *learned* through the kind of socialisation processes described by Dalton. Through therapy and meditation, Dalton gradually learned to re-connect with his emotions, as discussed in later chapters. Until then though, he felt he had been *'conditioned'* to disconnect from his emotions.

> *I remember the Cure had a hit with 'Boys don't cry'. I remember it meaning quite a lot to me at the time. I kind of made that connection, 'Oh yeah, I'm not supposed to cry.' [It wasn't] until I started therapy [that I was] really able to cry. Beforehand I'd only really done it [around] girlfriends, and then I'd always felt like it had come out of nowhere, I was always a bit embarrassed, or ashamed ... It's like I've got quite a bit of conditioning to not recognise these things.*

Disconnection from one's inner world

Thus, we come to the fourth main issue connected to masculinity: disconnection from one's inner world. We have seen that traditional masculine expectations created a climate where men came to view aspects of their being – particularly emotions around vulnerability and sadness – as unacceptable. Consequently, many men tried to repress or disconnect from these aspects. Unfortunately, the effect was to disconnect men from their emotional world. This confirms work by Addis (2008), whose gendered responding framework details how masculine norms influence the way men respond to emotions. '[R]estrictive norms defining how men should think, feel and behave' – especially the prescription to be emotionally tough – mean men are liable to disconnect from their emotions (p. 157). This framework was influenced by Nolen-Hoeksema's (1991) response-styles theory, which outlined gendered differences in emotional behaviour, including the notion that men have tendencies towards 'restrictive emotionality'. Nolen-Hoeksema's original theory tended towards an essentialist perspective, referring to 'sex-differences'. In contrast, drawing on social learning theory, Addis suggested socialisation pressures encouraged particular forms of gendered responding.

This disconnection had various deleterious consequences for participants here. First, many depicted their interiority as unfamiliar terrain.
Quite simply, they did not know themselves. Men portrayed a sense of
inner confusion, a decentred and chaotic subjectivity. Moreover, this
confusion was compounded by changing expectations of masculinity
as men grew into adulthood. As boys and teens, participants encountered traditional norms (e.g., toughness). These created conflict between
acceptable and unacceptable aspects of the self, as detailed above. However, this conflict became more complicated as hegemonic masculinity
itself shifted as men moved into new social arenas. Dalton described traditional norms as a *'set of rules'* about how he was *'supposed to be'* as a
man. In adulthood, some men found these 'rules' becoming challenged
and amended. For instance, Michael later socialised within feminist
circles, with differing expectations of masculinity to other settings –
different notions of 'acceptable' and 'unacceptable'. Some forms of feminism seek to amend inequalities in gender relations by encouraging the
emergence of the 'emotionally-expressive New Man' (Messner, 1993).
Michael followed this route, and tried to become *'this sensitive New Agey
man'*. However, this created new conflicts.

> *I was an anti-male feminist, trying to feminise myself, which was positively
> unhelpful. It meant I had a much darker shadow side, which didn't come
> out. Not allowing myself to know it, feeling guilty. [It] left too much of
> me out.*

Thus, traditional norms created an inner conflict between aspects of
self that aligned with these norms (acceptable) and those that contravened these (unacceptable). Encountering new sets of norms produced
a new conflict. These shifting expectations of masculinity created a sense
of identity confusion, as the original conflict became compounded by
other conflicts. Participants described the fragmentary experience of
not successfully negotiating multiple social contexts, each of which
appeared to require different gendered performances. Some suggested
they tried to adapt their behaviour to suit the context, leaving them
wondering which performance was the 'real' version of themselves. This
complicated their sense of internal conflict, and men described *'fragmentation'* or a *'lack of integration'*. Narratives here echo the work of
the constructionist identity theorist Gergen (2001), who challenges the
idea of a singular identity. Instead, he argues that our sense of self is
composed from multiple fragmentary 'small selves', a condition he calls
'multiphrenia'. For example, William was *'blokey'* with male friends who

wanted '*somebody to get pissed with*'; a '*good listener*' and a '*shoulder to cry on*' for female friends; with colleagues, '*professional*' and '*serious*'. The way his identity seemed to shift according to context and expectations left him confused.

> *I'd think, 'What am I? Who am I?' Utterly lost, a different person for different people ... liked by a lot of people, but because I was revealing to them only ... the bit they connected with. There would be all these different bits of me ... I used to feel like I didn't have very much inside me.*

Thus, in sum, various factors meant many men developed a problematic relationship with their interiority: they had been encouraged to disconnect from their emotions; societal norms meant aspects of the self were experienced as 'unacceptable', and were subject to repression; finally, *changes* in societal norms meant these conflicts became more complicated, and left men confused and fragmented. As a result, many men portrayed their inner world as a chaotic maelstrom over which they lacked control. The word '*turmoil*' was used by many to depict this state. Their narratives betrayed a sense of powerlessness, of being the victim of potent inner emotional forces that raged in spite of, or more accurately *because* of, men's attempts to disconnect from them. As William put it, '*I was completely oblivious to my internal processes ... going with whatever was happening, rather than aware of anything ... following one impulse after the other ... I was chaotic, no structure to my being.*' Here the narratives support the psychoanalytic argument that attempts to repress or disconnect from one's emotions and impulses do not make these disappear; instead they lurk out of sight and exert a malign influence of which the person is at best dimly aware. Some men depicted constant battles against inner forces they struggled to comprehend.

> *The waves chopped ... Rather than any sense of steering my boat, the wind took me ... Most of my life has been survival mode.* (Dustin)

This lack of control over a chaotic inner world was uncomfortable enough; it was particularly disturbing when the contents of this world were *negative*, as men became buffeted around by their distress. Men's narratives of powerlessness were most vivid as they recalled experiences of distress, a distress exacerbated by their inability to deal with it. Dalton: '*I had a lot of anger ... I didn't know what to do with it. Nobody taught me how to deal with my emotions ... You don't learn that at school.*' Moreover, men were intensely frustrated by their inability to deal with this distress, which served to compound the sense of turmoil. Anger/frustration in relation to lack of control was linked to self-destructive behaviours. Some described inviting destruction upon themselves. For instance, Ali recalled going *'off the rails'* after his marriage ended: *'I got into fights, nearly got stabbed...I was, "bring it on". It was anger at myself.'* Similarly, Henry recalled taking wild risks – *'playing with fire'* – in response to his turmoil, including *'dangerous games'*, like riding his motorbike with his eyes closed. It was not that he wanted to die per se, but his turmoil generated a reckless indifference to whether he lived.

> *There was no possibility for me to offload or let out steam...There was a strong need for the turmoil to stop. It wasn't about killing myself. I just wanted to stop it because I can't take it anymore.*

Men's narratives here powerfully demonstrate some important concepts in the literature on men's mental health. The debate on gendered differences in mental health is complicated. On the surface, the mental health of women appears worse than men. Women appear nearly twice as likely to experience common mental disorders as men (McManus et al., 2009). This trend is complicated by other factors. For example, gender intersects with ethnicity in complex ways: Irish and Pakistani men tend to fare worse than other men in terms of mental health, while Indian women seem to be worse off (Weich et al., 2004). Gender also intersects with age: depression is more common in women than men for people aged under 55, but after this age, this gender imbalance is reversed (Bebbington et al., 1998). Thus the intersectionality paradigm stresses the importance of considering how gender is affected by other factors, as explained above. However, intersectionality notwithstanding, higher rates of common mental disorders in women, particularly depression, are considered to be 'one of the most widely documented findings in psychiatric epidemiology' (Kessler, 2003, p. 6).

However, other alarming figures give cause for concern, suggesting men may experience and express distress and depression in other ways. For example, men are three times more likely to commit suicide than women (ONS, 2013), and constitute two out of every three deaths from alcohol (ONS, 2012b). Accounting for these trends, theorists suggest that rather than 'internalising' distress as sadness, as women are thought more prone to, men are more likely to 'externalise' it in various ways, including anger, aggression, risk-taking, substance/alcohol use, over-work and suicide (Pollack, 1998). As shown in the excerpts above, these are indeed the kind of behaviours men here were liable to undertake in response to distress. Researchers are beginning to recognise this pattern of externalising behaviours as a common response to distress among men. However, there are various interpretations as to what this means vis-à-vis the traditional diagnostic categories of mental illness. Here, discussions can become quite abstract, as scholars debate what we *mean* by concepts such as depression.

So far I have used the word 'distress' to cover the range of negative feelings experienced by men, from anger to 'turmoil'. As noted in Chapter 1, distress is a somewhat vague term used to denote negative experiences that fall short of clinical diagnoses for disorders. In contrast, defined illness categories have specific meanings. For example, major depressive disorder is diagnosed if five or more of the following symptoms persist for two weeks: depressed mood, diminished interest in pleasure, weight loss, sleep disturbance, psychomotor agitation, energy loss, feelings of guilt or worthlessness, diminished ability to think/concentrate, and recurrent thoughts of death (APA, 2013). Some gender theorists argue that these generic diagnostic criteria reflect the 'internalising' responses seemingly favoured by women, like rumination, a diagnostic bias which is seen as explaining the *apparently* lower rates of depression in men (Kilmartin, 2005). The externalising behaviours commonly exhibited by men in response to distress, like anger or suicidality, are not included within these criteria. This has led to debate over what we *should* call this pattern of behaviours. Addis (2008) distinguishes between two different frameworks with subtly different interpretations: the masked depression framework and the masculine depression framework.

The masked depression framework (e.g., Cochran & Rabinowitz, 2000) suggests that men do experience 'prototypic' depression, corresponding to conventional diagnostic criteria, such as depressed mood. However, men are frequently unable to *recognise* this in themselves, as they have been encouraged by traditional masculine norms to 'distract, avoid, or get angry in the presence of negative affect' (Addis, 2008, p. 161). Thus, although men may *feel* depressed, as conventionally understood, their depression is hidden, or 'masked', both from themselves and from others. Men's inability to recognise it in themselves connects to the idea of alexithymia. In terms of masking it from others too, men are generally seen as reluctant to admit to distress and seek help, a reluctance linked to norms of invulnerability and toughness (Addis & Mahalik, 2003). Indeed, we will see in the next chapter that participants were often unwilling to seek help for their problems, doing so only when they had reached crisis point. Moreover, even if men do seek help, people may only see the 'presenting symptoms' (e.g., anger), and not discern the underlying 'depression' and distress (Rabinowitz & Cochran, 2008).

The masculine depression framework approaches the externalising behaviours in a different way, suggesting that these constitute a 'phenotypic variant of prototypic depression' (Addis, 2008, p. 159). Here, it is not that men experience depression as conventionally understood (e.g., depressed mood) but express this in unique ways (e.g., anger). Rather, it is argued that men are liable to a distinct 'male-specific' form of depression which *involves* feelings like anger. The narratives here uphold both frameworks. Some men did describe having depressed feelings, but getting frustrated by their inability to deal with these, which led to feelings of anger (as per the masked depression framework). For other men, their distress took the *form* of anger, which was compounded by their lack of coping skills (as per the masculine depression framework). Either way, many participants described being at the mercy of their negative feelings. We can see that learning to disconnect from emotions did not render men emotionless; on the contrary, their emotions continued to rage, sometimes violently so. Having disconnected though, men were often powerless victims to these feelings. Learning to manage their emotional world proved to be one of the benefits of meditation that men valued the most. Until then though, many men experienced a torrid time.

> *I was always battling, I had suicidal thoughts. It comes out of a sense you've got nowhere to go with your mindset. Internal stuff was so strongly negative, it would be triggered and I would be, 'I want to be obliterated, I want to be annihilated, I don't want this pain, this emotional pain.'* (Colin)

Summary

Growing up, participants encountered traditional masculine norms around toughness. These exerted a particularly powerful effect as participants crossed a threshold from boyhood to manhood in early adolescence. Participants generally sought to enact these norms, partly out of concern with fitting in, partly as a way of coping with vulnerability. However, this led to adverse consequences. Men experienced a destructive inner conflict between aspects of the self deemed acceptable and aspects deemed unacceptable. As a result, men tried to repress or disconnect from these unacceptable aspects. Consequently, many men became detached from their emotional life. This had the unfortunate consequence that men found it difficult to deal with distress, which often became 'externalised', e.g., in the form of anger and suicidality. The next chapter explores some of the ways in which men did try to deal with their feelings – ways which were ultimately experienced as unsuccessful – before showing how participants eventually turned to meditation as a solution to their problems.

3
Seeking Wellbeing

> *I'd gone through a really tough period of time, personally,*
> *emotionally, career wise, nearly lost absolutely everything...I came*
> *to meditation as a means of wanting to find space and calmness in*
> *what at that time was a maelstrom.* (Dustin)

In the last chapter, we saw that participants encountered traditional masculine norms around toughness as they were growing up. As a result, many men became disconnected from their emotions, which meant they often struggled to deal with their feelings of distress. However, it was not that men did not *try* to deal with these feelings. This chapter begins by exploring the different ways in which men tried to pursue wellbeing. Unfortunately, these ways ultimately were experienced as unsuccessful. Consequently, men eventually turned to meditation in the hope of finding a better way to attain wellbeing, as set out in the second part of the chapter.

Trying (unsuccessfully) to find wellbeing

In their stories of life before they found meditation, participants gave the impression of being engaged in a forlorn and ultimately futile pursuit, seeking wellbeing in ways that ultimately proved unsuccessful. I do not mean to imply that all men were searching for the same thing. Some were searching for pleasure, others for meaning, many for relief from distress, and most for 'happiness', in whatever way they chose to define this. However, as elucidated in Chapter 1, wellbeing is a multidimensional term that encompasses all these facets. Thus I will speak here generally of participants searching for wellbeing, though I will try to also give a sense of the specific aspects of wellbeing that different people were searching for. Whatever men *were* looking for, there were four main places they turned to: romantic relationships; drink and drugs; work and material rewards; and hobbies. We might refer to these here as 'remedies' for wellbeing. Most men looked in hope – and ultimately in vain – to some, if not all, of these remedies for their wellbeing. As Andrew said: *'Take drugs, drink, possess things, people, relationship, career, whatever.'* There was also a fifth remedy that many men would have *liked to* have been able to turn to, but felt unable to: religion. This section looks at these remedies in turn, exploring the hope men invested in them, and the ways in which they finally let men down.

Relationships

In the previous chapter, we saw that participants were influenced by masculinity norms that demanded that they be tough. Consequently, men often adopted a hyperagentic 'lone man' stance, becoming disconnected from others. The friendships men did have were portrayed as lacking depth, and men generally felt unable to open up emotionally to friends. However, there was one important exception to this pattern of disconnection: romantic relationships. These were the one place that men felt able to 'let their guard down'. That is not to say that men abandoned all concern with traditional norms around their romantic partners – men still described hiding their emotions sometimes, or feeling the need to be strong. Yet at the same time, the 'private' arena of romantic relationships offered something of a sanctuary from the more onerous requirements of the public realm in terms of attaining hegemonic masculinity. In the context of such relationships, men reported a complex dynamic, partly upholding traditional norms, but also partly relinquishing these and letting a softer, more vulnerable side emerge, as Allen (2007) also found. Thus, relationships allowed men at least *the chance* to loosen up some of their rigidity around how they were as men.

> *I needed to meet her for her to show me the way and to broaden my horizons…She made me look at life a bit bigger and I needed that, it was a great thing.* (Alvin)

In this context, men frequently described turning towards romantic relationships for their emotional needs. Other scholars have suggested that heterosexual men tend to 'downplay' the importance of romance in their life, partly out of concern with meeting traditional hegemonic norms around self-sufficiency (Gilmartin, 2007). However, I found that men of all sexual orientations were very open about the importance of romantic liaisons in their lives before meditation (after starting meditation, these diminished somewhat in importance). Across the narratives was a panoply of reasons that men valued their romantic relationships. Some men focused on their positive rewards. Michael mentioned feeling good (*'Love ... makes you feel wonderful'*), while Sam highlighted sexual excitement (*'We stirred up lots of energy'*). A common theme was turning to relationships as a solution to emotional problems, hoping that relationships would *'take care'* of these. We can see this hope as a counterpart to the lack of control men had over their emotional world, as set out in Chapter 2. Lacking the ability to manage their own emotional problems, men nursed a hope that being in a relationship would somehow be a solution.

> *I knew that I wasn't in a happy life, [but] I thought a relationship would sort that out [and] allow me to be happy.* (Colin)

It is important to recognise that when relationships were flourishing, they really did seem to ameliorate men's emotional problems. For example, Ross spoke about yearning to overcome the *'pain of being a separate person'*, and that when he was in a successful relationship, he did indeed find the emotional connection he was looking for. Similarly, Silas found *'security'* in monogamy. However, and most crucially, the wellbeing men gained from relationships was 'precarious', as it was contingent on the success of the relationship. Unfortunately, most narratives on relationships were about these *failing*. Here, the consequent distress became a bigger part of their narrative than the positive impact of the relationship. The most acute narratives of distress were invariably linked to relationship break-ups. In this sense, *relying* on relationships to ameliorate emotional issues was not only ineffectual but could actually be counter-productive. A number of men discussed suicidality linked to relationship troubles. For example, William had hoped that relationships would offer a solution to his unhappiness: *'I was looking for the one person I could put all my hopes on and we'd live together forever and it would be blissful.'* Whenever these relationships failed, he was distraught.

> *[Whenever] it didn't work out I'd be absolutely crushed, feeling suicidal. I used to think, 'Do I have anything inside me holding me together?' I'd be utterly bereft ... just this cold nothingness inside ... literally like you don't have a heart.*

Drink and drugs

Many men turned to alcohol and psychoactive substances as a solution to their problems. It is recognised that drink and drugs are problems for men. In England and Wales, men account for around two out of every three deaths from both alcohol (ONS, 2012a) and illicit drugs (ONS, 2012c). We see various explanations for these trends. Males are more likely to be offered drink and drugs, and from a younger age, than females (Moon et al., 1999). It is also argued that drinking and taking drugs are prominent ways for men to perform masculinity, i.e., men demonstrate their manhood by being able to 'handle' their drink (de Visser & Smith, 2007). However, the narratives here offer a different reason, one that may seem obvious but is often overlooked in the literature: drink/drugs were valued for having the capacity to change one's *emotional state*. That drink/drugs are often described as 'psychoactive' – i.e., 'affecting the mind or mood or other mental processes' – is especially pertinent here. We saw in Chapter 2 that men often had trouble engaging with their interior world, and lacked control over their emotions. In this context, the value of drink/drugs was that they seemed to offer men a way of directly altering their emotional state.

As we shall see, the psychoactive effects of drink/drugs were often unpredictable, and men came to view these as an unstable and ultimately destructive route to emotional management. However, at least at first, men experienced drink/drugs as an effective shortcut to wellbeing. Some men highlighted their pleasurable effects: Jack was attracted to the hedonistic potential of drugs (*'Intensifying experience with pleasure'*); Terry described how marijuana initially enabled a sense of freedom (*'Euphoric ... more creative, more light'*). These stories echo a study on university students which found that the overwhelming reason given for using drink/drugs was the pursuit of pleasure (Webb et al., 1996). In contrast, other men described the positive effect of drink/drugs on wellbeing in terms of their ability to ameliorate emotional issues. For example, Ross used substances to overcome his feelings of isolation and disconnectedness from others (*'Relief from the pain of being a separate somebody'*). Lacking skills to engage with emotions effectively, substances became an indirect way of regulating emotional states. Terry recalled the initial success of this strategy.

> *[I had] really difficult times with my mental state, depression, stress, anxiety. My self-medication was smoking far too much dope. It's hardly surprising I became hooked because it was such a strong, marked difference from how I felt a lot of the time, an easy quick fix to all the neuroses, all the pain I was carrying around.*

However, most men suggested that, ultimately, self-medication with alcohol/substances was a 'maladaptive' emotional management strategy. For example, Silas described using drugs to blunt and *'suppress'* negative feelings (*'A subduing effect on the emotional life'*). His story reflects a prominent idea in the literature on masculinity and mental health; namely, that men are prone to the kind of 'avoidant' coping strategies outlined in Chapter 1. That is, influenced by masculine norms around toughness and emotional disconnection – as detailed above – men are liable to 'avoid' contact with their own feelings of distress. In this sense, trying to blunt distress with drink/drugs is a classic avoidance response (Labouvie & Bates, 2002).

Unfortunately, men's stories here also reflected another idea that is well-recognised in this literature: dissociating from emotions became a problematic way of dealing with them. Silas recalled how *'suppression'* with drugs left him feeling *'disconnect[ed]'*. Moreover, self-medication failed to keep his issues at bay: the emotion eventually *'catches up'*, and *'what's repressed breaks through'*. His story echoes the psychoanalytic perspective on repression outlined above, where repressed material continues to exert a malign influence. Both Silas and Terry implicated substance use in breakdowns they subsequently experienced (see below). Thus, like relationships, drink/drugs were a 'precarious' solution to men's problems.

> *It works for a bit but then it starts to work less so you then need more for it to work in the same way. Then it starts to not work because it starts to actually exacerbate in the long term the problems that it was resolving... You get the come down and get all the paranoia and the neuroses, just bigger.*
> (Terry)

Work and rewards

A third area men looked to for wellbeing was their work, and/or the rewards that work could bring. Regarding work itself, most men recognised it had a functional dimension – earning money was necessary in order to maintain a standard of living. Indeed, for some men, their work represented nothing more than that (Grant: *'I really had to work to survive, because I didn't have any money'*). However, many men invested some hope in their careers, viewing these as a vocation that could offer meaning and fulfilment. Indeed, occupations are a potent source of PWB, particularly when they satisfy key requirements: for example, aligning with a person's core values; opportunities to experience positive emotions; and enabling the person to exercise some choice with regard to their daily activities (George & Jones, 1996). Some participants entered careers which they felt did align with their values, and would enable them to find meaning. For example, quite a few men overcame masculine pressures and took up a career that is traditionally regarded as 'feminine': nursing (Pullen & Simpson, 2009). These men saw this as a chance to enact the caring ideals they wanted to express, but were generally discouraged from doing in everyday life. Even though his father *'very much wanted me to do something else'*, Silas was attracted to nursing.

> *I had a moment of vision on my bed, as a 16 year old, that I just wanted to care for people, that that would be a very noble hope ... [I tried] a placement [and] really enjoyed it. It was about connecting with someone in a much more simple way ... just being with people.*

However, for many men, their stories about work often centred on how these had failed to provide a sense of wellbeing. For men whose work was purely functional – i.e., they did not see it as a vocation – there was a palpable sense that work was demoralising. For example, Alvin was disenchanted with being a cog in the machinery of a large company: *'They give you a salary and buy you a jumper with the company logo, but in return they take your bloody soul and your dignity and ... make you feel like a bag of shit.'* Indeed, a long line of thinkers stemming back to Karl Marx have argued that modern economic systems generate dehumanising work conditions, where individuals are fungible (replaceable) parts of a system geared to serve the interests of the few (Vincent, 1988). Even for men for whom work was a vocation, job demands were such that it was experienced more as a source of stress than fulfilment. This stress was related to an overbearing workload, and a diminishing assessment of one's capacity to manage this, as elucidated in the 'job demand–control model' (Karasek, 1997). For example, despite Silas's choosing nursing as a vocation – and initially experiencing it as rewarding as such – he *'started disengaging'* as work became over-demanding.

> *From a process of engaging, living from one's ideals, to a process of disengaging, [was] very painful. The sense of resentment, the sense of lack, really, an inability to respond in the way I used to. You could call it burnout.*

Many men had also hoped to find happiness through the rewards of work, socially in terms of status, and materialistically in terms of wealth and possessions. Social commentators often lament that materialism is the dominant ideology of modern Western society, the so-called age of 'consumerism', where our identity is defined by what we buy and possess (Campbell, 2004). Many participants agreed with this scathing assessment. Ali said he had been *'taught'* by his family, and by society, that wealth was *'what life is about'*, and that money had been his *'religion'*. Consequently, some men came to place a high value on monetary and material wealth, and thus had oriented their life around the pursuit of these rewards. A number of these men had indeed been successful in this regard, entering well-remunerated occupations. However, these men reported that these did not provide the fulfilment they had hoped to find in them (John: *'It doesn't bring the happiness I think it [will]'*). The narratives echo findings around the hedonic treadmill, where beyond a certain point of comfort, extrinsic rewards like money are quickly acclimatised to, and do not enhance SWB. Thus, a number of men told a tale of ceasing to look to material rewards for their wellbeing. Alvin:

> *When I first started my business degree I wanted to be an investment banker, work in the City. I was attracted by the suits, the Porsche, the money. But from the experience of living in a block full of investment bankers, it's the last thing I want to do. They all had nice big cars, the nice apartment block with all the facilities, but they were all miserable as sin, the most miserable people I've ever met in my life.*

Hobbies

The fourth main area that men turned to in search of wellbeing was hobbies, particularly sport and artistic pursuits. Much of the literature on masculinity and sport focuses on the way that sporting arenas and contexts are vehicles for inculcating traditional masculine gender norms, e.g., reproducing and encouraging hegemonic behaviours like competitiveness and toughness (Parker, 2006). Indeed, narratives here did suggest that social environments around sporting participation were often suffused with a traditional masculine ethos, where men would engage in ostentatious displays of hyperagentic aggression. William's football team was full of *'blokey blokes'* who would *'shout at each other on the pitch, get into arguments with the referee, go down the pub afterwards and get pissed'*.

Participants generally disliked this ethos and resisted succumbing to it themselves. Crucially though, they valued their sporting hobby *in spite* of it. For example, despite the aggressive ethos, men nevertheless made good friends through their hobby, as other researchers have found (Harvey, 1999). In addition, though often overlooked within the masculinity literature, a large body of work has linked exercise to wellbeing: aside from any social benefits, it can increase SWB (Reed & Ones, 2006) and reduce distress (Hassmén et al., 2000). For example, Kris really enjoyed playing cricket, not for the feeling of winning, but for the pleasure of participating.

> *My theory was, playing's not about winning, playing's about having a good time and improving as cricketers. That's all we can do.*

Men also appreciated sport for another reason, a reason which also applied to artistic hobbies – the chance to experience 'flow'. As outlined in Chapter 1, flow refers to a state in which attention is entirely focused on the task at hand, which then serves to diminish people's sense of self and awareness of time (Csikszentmihalyi, 1990). From a psychological perspective, flow is theorised as the third main type of wellbeing, in addition to SWB and PWB. Together, these constitute the 'good life', comprising the engaged life (flow), the pleasurable life (SWB) and the meaningful life (PWB) (Seligman, 2002). Men described experiencing flow (not that men themselves used this term) across a diverse range of activities, from playing the guitar (Dean: *'I loved losing myself in music'*) and the piano (Robert: *'Consciousness is absorbed on one thing, it becomes contemplative'*) to dancing (Ernest: *'Peace in a very energetic state'*). Some suggested that this state of absorption was an early precursor of a mental stillness they would later come to appreciate in meditation. Kris on cricket:

> *It's a unique game, it requires a lot of focus and attention and a lot of mindfulness ... especially being a batsman ... because things happen quickly but they're very spaced out ... I've loved that mental side of it.*

Men's narratives around their hobbies were generally very positive. In fact, these seemed to be men's most reliable source of wellbeing. Compared to the other 'remedies', hobbies were less likely to exacerbate men's issues (unlike drugs), generate undue stress (unlike work), or fail/end (unlike relationships). However, while hobbies were rewarding, men suggested that these had little impact upon wellbeing *outside* the activity. That is, the satisfaction derived from experiencing pleasure or flow whilst engaging in their hobby had a lingering afterglow, but this swiftly dissipated. Moreover, the time men were able to spend on such activities was often limited. A few participants tried to expand the role their favoured hobby had in their life by pursuing a career in it. Unfortunately though, doing so tended to lessen the contentment they derived from it, since it introduced other dimensions to the activity which detracted from their enjoyment. For example, Robert hated the *'business side'* of trying to earn money from piano playing, while Michael's artistic passion *'died'* in the competitive environment of art school. Moreover, some said that, while enjoyable, their hobby struggled to satisfy a deeper sense of wellbeing.

> *[I] always expected being in bands and stuff like that to give me some sort of sense of fulfilment...It's fun, but it isn't an ultimate meaning.* (Dean)

Religion

Finally, there was an area that men were *unable* to turn to for their wellbeing needs: religion. The reason this warrants mentioning is that religion featured prominently in men's narratives of youth as something many *wanted* to turn to, but could not. The majority of participants had been raised in religious families, usually Christian, and most had fond memories of childhood experiences of religion. This fondness generally pertained to its social aspects. For example, Grant recalled his church feeling *'like a family, a sense of not being isolated'*. However, all those raised as religious were compelled to walk away from it, usually in the threshold period of early adolescence, which is a common age for a loss of faith (Uecker et al., 2007). Generally, participants described ceasing to believe in the central tenets of the religion. As Peter put it, *'The basic theology I just never got on with...I was open to being convinced, [but it was] a leap of faith that I couldn't make.'* There were various reasons given for this erosion of belief. Peter attributed this to his *'scientific background'*. William wrestled with the troubling idea of eternal damnation.

> *I did try [to believe]. God knows I had a go. But I knew by the time I was 14 that I was going through the motions. [I thought], 'Why would [God] give you 70 years to be good and if you screw up then you're damned for eternity.' That doesn't sound to me like a God who's full of love, it sounds like a God who's a bit of a psychopath. And I couldn't ever get a really good answer on that.*

Thus, some participants rejected religious beliefs after subjecting these to rational analysis. (As we shall see, upon taking up meditation, many men became attracted to Buddhism. Its ability to win their rational assent, rather than commanding a leap of faith, was an important factor in this attraction.) Another reason for rejecting religion was a social atmosphere that was perceived to be judgemental. Some men experienced their religious community as hostile to outsiders. For example,

Ali was raised a Hindu, and his decision to marry a non-Hindu woman caused a schism within his family and the wider community (*'A tragedy, I couldn't tell my dad he had two grandchildren'*). Particularly problematic, given the high number of gay participants, was the issue of homophobia, a common problem in religious communities, especially more conservative ones (Finlay & Walther, 2003). (Although Buddhism is not exempt from homophobia (Scherer, 2011), it is often relatively accepting of homosexuality (Schalow, 1992), which was a factor in its appeal here.) Grant had already rejected religion in adolescence; however, an experience in adulthood after the death of his partner, where his partner's church did not want to let him attend the funeral, was particularly galling.

> *I had a terrible tussle after [my partner] died with the church ... who didn't want the queer mafia in their church. They didn't really want him in, or want us in ... I had no faith before that [anyway, but] that put me off the Christians rather badly.*

However, there were notable differences in the subsequent impact that rejection of religion had on men's journey to meditation. Prior to taking up meditation, most participants saw it as 'spiritual' in some way. Thus, men's willingness to engage with meditation depended to an extent on how they saw the relationship between spirituality and religion. Scholars usually use 'religion' to refer to social institutions centred around particular beliefs, practices and rituals. In contrast, 'spirituality' is rather vaguer, i.e., 'something individuals define for themselves that is largely free of the rules, regulations and responsibilities associated with religion' (Hasanović et al., 2011, p. 331). Some men saw spirituality as different to religion. Despite rejecting religion, these men had remained open to spirituality, searching for outlets for their spiritual feelings. For example, Michael recalled thinking: *'"I'll pop into a church, but I don't quite know why", even though I didn't believe in God.'* As explored below, these men found meditation relatively early in adult life, and embraced it easily. Other men had conflated religion with spirituality: rejection of religion hindered their engagement with spirituality. Consequently, this resistance to spirituality meant these men usually had greater difficulty eventually engaging with meditation.

> *I didn't regard myself as spiritual ... I saw meditation in that bracket ... I thought it was synonymous with religion, and I very much regarded myself as an atheist.* (Silas)

With this excerpt, we move into the second part of this chapter. This examines the different reasons men finally turned to meditation, and the various ways in which they did so. Men who were resistant to spirituality had a harder time countenancing meditation – their route was harder, and often involved serious emotional issues. Thus as we shall see, men differed in terms of how easily and how early in life they were able to find meditation, which had significant implications for their wellbeing.

Turning to meditation

We have seen that although men had difficulties managing their emotions, they nevertheless pursued wellbeing through various 'remedies', notably relationships, drink/drugs, work and hobbies. Here, we will see that men turned to meditation when they came to the conclusion that these remedies were incapable of addressing their needs, and that something else would be needed. Interestingly, most participants were *aware* of the existence of meditation in their early adulthood, if not before. Some discovered it from family members (Grant: '*My father had an interest in Eastern religions [that] filtered down to us kids*'). Others just knew about it from its general cultural presence, e.g, as part of the 1960s counterculture (Harry: '*It was all part of the love, hippy, slightly druggy haze*'). However, men's narratives about turning to meditation concerned how this awareness of meditation shifted into the feeling that it was something they wanted to try *for themselves*. There were four main reasons men turned to meditation: exploring different 'ways of being'; in response to stress; after a period of existential questioning; and following a breakdown. As will become clear, these reasons represented predicaments of escalating levels of 'seriousness' – those who found meditation through the first reason had a relatively easy journey; those who only turned to it following a breakdown had a much harder route.

Exploring different ways of being

A small minority of participants began meditating in their early twenties, if not earlier. These men were not only ahead of the curve in terms of finding meditation, they were exceptions to many of the themes discussed so far: they did not generally succumb to traditional masculine norms; they were less detached from their inner world, with fewer difficulties managing emotions; and they rarely pursued wellbeing through the remedies above. In fact, these men's stories offer clues on how many of the issues highlighted so far might be ameliorated or even avoided.

Their narratives shared various characteristics. First, these men high-lighted a keen sense of curiosity in childhood, and indicated that their engagement with meditation stemmed directly from it. For example, Robert was fascinated by magic as a child ('*I saw my first show at five. I couldn't believe it, excitement, awe, wonder*'), leading to an interest in '*the occult*' and the '*Western mystery traditions*'. He met older practition-ers of magic and theosophy, who introduced him to meditation aged 15. Others recalled formative incidents which awakened their curiosity, and which were early precursors of meditative-type experiences. Peter recalled a day in childhood as '*the first time I learned...I could affect my mind*'.

> *I was in a bad mood, and thought, 'I'll take myself off for a walk in the woods', and came back feeling good. It was then it clicked that I could change my mental state.*

A second quality this minority shared was an independent streak. Compared to others, these men seemed more immune to hegemonic pressures. When they discussed the threshold to manhood, rather than focusing on vulnerability and toughness, or a concern with fitting in, these men were more likely to emphasise themes of freedom and non-conformity. This takes us back to the importance of upbringing, outlined in Chapter 1. In particular, most of these 'non-conforming' men sug-gested their independence had been encouraged by a 'facilitative' family environment which encouraged exploration. For example, as already discussed, Sam moved into a community of vegetarians as a teenager, supported by his parents: '*They found it important I live my life the way I wanted...My conscience was awoken.*'

However, it is important to note that this narrative of independence was not always presented in a positive light. A few men felt that the corollary of being relatively resistant to social pressures was a degree of isolation. In later chapters, we will see how most men eventually became involved with communities of other people who shared their interest in meditation. However, until then, in pursing their inter-ests alone, some recalled disconnection from peers. Unlike Sam, whose independence was channelled in positive ways by his family, Robert depicted a dysfunctional upbringing. He was alienated in pursuing his independence as a young man.

> *I just wasn't involved in the normal, the usual, the conventional...I had a peer group but I didn't belong to it, not at school nor anywhere...Friends*

> *used to find me odd ... I didn't find it easy ... I was often on my own [and]*
> *very lonely, but I had to follow my passions.*

These men indicated that their sense of independence and curiosity was partly responsible for them finding meditation. They presented a narrative of rejecting what they regarded as a conventional path, e.g., concern with materialism. Instead, they sought to determine their own values and work out their own priorities, exploring alternative ways of being. These men were philosophically engaged, often interested in humanism and existentialism, and were pre-occupied with seeking meaning in life. From an existential point of view, these young men embarked on a 'quest for meaning' (Wong & Fry, 1998). Many participants would not become concerned with this until later in life (see below). Indeed, Merriam and Heuer (1996) suggest that some people do not embark on this quest at all. Through their explorations of alternative ways of being, these men moved in countercultural circles and soon encountered meditation. Meditation was recalled as immediately intriguing, a possible source of the meaning they had sought. More specifically, these men's interest was especially piqued by the Buddhist context in which they encountered meditation. While these men had rejected religion, they remained open to spirituality. They were unsure whether Buddhism *was* a religion – interestingly, this ambiguity was never clearly resolved, as discussed in later chapters. Nevertheless, Buddhism seemed sufficiently different to previous experiences of religion to command their interest.

> *I've always had a strong desire for meaning in my life from an early age ...*
> *I was very keen to go to university, more for meeting new people, explo-*
> *ration. When I was there, I had a group of friends who were ... influenced*
> *by Sartre and the idea that you have to create your own meaning ... I even-*
> *tually met someone ... who was a Buddhist ... It really fitted in, 'OK, so*
> *this is a potential tool for meaning.'*

Unfortunately, most men did not have the inclination or the opportunity to pursue alternative ways of being in this way. They became drawn into a more conventional existence, searching (in vain) for wellbeing through the remedies above. Their journey towards meditation was more arduous and complicated.

Responding to stress

Most men did not have the fortune or the adventurousness to find meditation in their early adulthood. Instead, they tried to pursue wellbeing and manage their emotional issues through the 'remedies' – relationships, drink/drugs, work and hobbies. Unfortunately, these remedies were found to be at best limited, and at worst counterproductive, as elucidated above. In light of these limitations, some men managed to turn to meditation as a better way of dealing with their stress/distress. The crucial consideration here is why only *some* men managed to do this. Unlike those in the first 'group' who found meditation through exploration of other ways of being, these men had not explicitly sought a different way of life. However, they were open-minded and amenable to trying something alternative like meditation if the opportunity came up and the circumstances were right.

Some had already dabbled with meditation previously, e.g., at university. However, unlike the men who embraced meditation early in life, this initial interest was not followed up. One reason was that financial concerns prevented them indulging in the pursuit of alternative ways of being. This finding is important, since it shows that embarking on an early quest for meaning is not simply a question of 'character', where only some men are viewed as having the 'inner-directed' inclination to pursue their own path, as Riesman and colleagues (1961) suggested. Rather, it shows how socio-economic factors play a strong (though not inevitable) determining role in the paths people are *allowed* by their circumstances to take. Some of those who pursued an early interest in spirituality, described above, indicated that this had been helped by a favourable socio-economic background; this provided them with the means and the safety to take a risk, to indulge a youthful idealism and strike out on unconventional paths. As Peter said: *'[I had a] very stable background. It was like, "What am I going to do with this life? I've got an opportunity here".'* As others have found, being able to construct and pursue an idiosyncratic 'lifestyle' is a luxury that may not be open to those from more impoverished backgrounds (Veal, 1993). Some men here said that having time and space to explore meditation depended upon a degree of financial security they lacked at the time.

> *We were young and poor, starting our careers. There wasn't an awful lot of parental financial support. You had to make your own way as quickly as you could. I had to concentrate on making a living, so a lot of things were quietly forgotten until I had a bit more space.* (Grant)

A second reason for not pursuing an early interest in meditation relates to a broader theme that ran through most narratives: it fell outside patterns of behaviour encouraged by traditional hegemonic masculinity.

Many indicated that taking up meditation went against social norms, and meant stepping outside their circle of friends. Unlike the more independent men above, most men had difficulties challenging expectations; thus, this was a barrier to engagement, which many found hard to overcome. For example, despite wanting to try meditation, Dalton put off going to a class for over a year: *'Going to a Buddhist centre felt quite alternative . . . Nobody I knew meditated. All my mates just wanted to go down the pub and drink.'* As such, men often faced considerable social pressure not to engage in meditation, as it transgressed expectations around masculinity. Moreover, irrespective of gender, many men felt meditation was viewed with suspicion by society generally – i.e., meditators of both sexes were regarded strangely, not only male meditators. Alvin felt there was a *'stigma'* attached to it: *'People look at you like, "he's a bit cuckoo".'* This kind of stigma put some men off meditating. Harry had enrolled for a meditation course at university years ago. His wariness about meditation as *'esoteric stuff'* was compounded by *'powerful disapprovals'* from his family.

> *It was all too scary . . . I didn't have anybody else who was interested in it . . . to have a discussion or to normalise it in any way . . . There were several elements that made it fearful . . . There was the drug culture of the 60's that was hanging over . . . I was drawn between being a teenager and wanting those current age things, and at the same time having strong messages within which says, 'This is dangerous.'*

Lacking peer support to help him overcome this wariness, Harry didn't attend the course. His interest in meditation *'sank beneath the waves'*. Having flirted with the notion of travelling a less conventional path, exploring a more 'spiritual' way of being, he *'put all that away till later'*, becoming *'rigidly scientific'*. Thus we can see how a nascent attraction to meditation was snubbed out, when with some social encouragement it might have flowered sooner. As it was, Harry didn't return to meditation until 20 years later. There were three main factors in this return. First, with age and independence came the assertiveness to resist social pressures that previously impeded him. Indeed, theorists of psychological development contend that increasing age is often accompanied by greater individuation – the shaping of 'character' in maturity (Markus & Herzog, 1991). Second, meditation itself was becoming more normalised in the 1970s and 1980s as practices such as Transcendental Meditation (TM) were presented in less contentious terms as 'relaxation techniques' (Benson et al., 1974). Third, and most crucially, was the proximate *factor* that prompted Harry to return to meditation. As we shall see, it is common in men's stories to find that a particular event was a dramatic 'tipping point' that compelled men to take action to change. Harry had flourished in a stressful business career for years, but was compelled to return to meditation as a way of coping with the *'trauma and impact'* of a partner being diagnosed with a terminal illness.

> *It was, 'How do you hold your life together and deal with the stress and anxiety at the same time as getting on with your life?' I had a high powered job, so in those days my intention to meditate was entirely to do with stress management.*

Some other participants also turned to meditation as a better way of managing stress/distress. However, for these men, this was not a case of returning to meditation having previously put off engagement with it. Instead these participants, who were mostly younger men, described 'stumbling' on meditation or Buddhism, usually whilst travelling around Asia. These men had generally set off, not intending to explore Buddhism/meditation, but in pursuit of fun and adventure. For example, Ernest was *'seeking pleasure and hedonism, girls, weed, beaches, escapism from anything I had back home'*. As Ernest's statement suggests, some men also travelled to get away from their troubles, borne by the vague sense that life might be better elsewhere. Indeed, scholars have interpreted the modern phenomenon of 'backpacking' as a form of migratory lifestyle centred around the search for a better way of life (Cohen, 2011). Abroad, men encountered Buddhism through visiting temples or imbibing the atmosphere of a Buddhist society. Many were *'intrigued'* by Buddhist images, discourses and attitudes they came across. In particular, men were curious about the possibility that there were other ways of attaining wellbeing than the strategies they were currently using (Ernest: *'The promise of peace was something which piqued my interest'*). Men tended to depict these experiences overseas as turning points in their stories. Alvin had his own version of the 'tipping point':

> *I was pumping a lot of weights, doing a lot of drugs... The reason I went travelling is I had been charged for the second time [with a driving offence]... nearly killed lots of people... Life was becoming so wild that my father said to me... 'Go to Thailand and calm down'. ... It was the biggest turning point of my life... I left an aggressive, self-important, pumped-up, stupid, thoughtless, careless, uncaring person... I come back completely in love with the world.*

Thus we have seen that some men began meditating early in adulthood through a pursuit of alternative ways of being, whilst other men turned to it slightly later as a way of dealing with stress/distress. However, the majority of men continued looking to the 'remedies' for their wellbeing, until some of these men began to question if these remedies were really *working*.

Existential questioning

Some men turned to meditation following a difficult period of existential questioning. Unlike those above, these men had not sought an alternate way of being in early adulthood, nor had they stumbled upon one. Instead, they were drawn into a conventional existence structured around the remedies. That is, these participants were leading what many people might regard as a normal life in contemporary Western society: trying to forge careers and earn money, cultivating romantic relationships, engaging in hobbies, and indulging in regular drinking and occasional recreational drugs. The capacity of these remedies to deal with men's emotional problems and generate wellbeing fluctuated over time: at points, the remedies would fail, as outlined above; at other times, men felt these remedies were more successful, like when in the midst of a successful relationship, or if one's career was flourishing. However, for a number of men, a subtle but crucial shift in perspective began to occur. Rather than making judgements on how well they were 'playing the game' in terms of these remedies – whether they could be doing better in work, whether their particular relationship was working – they began to question the very remedies themselves.

> When I got through university and started work, I was just out getting pissed, taking loads of drugs, and chasing after women ... but I remember just feeling quite lost. My career was progressing but I remember just thinking, 'Is this it? Is this me? Is this what I've got to do in life? Because it doesn't feel like much at all.' (William)

As such, these men had a crisis of *meaning*. As elucidated in Chapter 1, finding meaning in life is central to PWB. However, 'meaning' is a subtle concept. Having a sense of meaning fulfils two important needs: for comprehensibility (a framework of beliefs that allows one to understand existence); and for significance (a sense that existence has purpose) (Janoff-Bulman & Yopyk, 2004). Moreover, meaning can be appraised both globally (in terms of life in general), and individually (in terms of one's own life) (Park, 2005). Given these different needs and forms of appraisal, there are various ways in which life could lack meaning. For example, one may possess a cognitive framework that renders existence comprehensible, e.g., a scientific theory of evolution, and yet still not feel one's *own* existence has significance. Or one could have a global sense of life having purpose, yet feel that one's day-to-day activities do not serve this purpose, such that the specific individual acts of one's life lack significance. In the narratives here, a lack of meaning was experienced in various ways. For example, a few said that, for as long as they could remember, they had been burdened by a vague, uneasy sense of the purposelessness of the existence they were brought into. Michael recalled feeling this even as a child, and had harboured '*nihilistic*' thoughts for a long time.

> *Part of my unhappiness was that I just thought, 'I don't believe this, it's just rubbish . . . this existence we all value, small little houses, families, church tombolas'. . . . I had a strong 'What's the point, it's all kind of crap' kind of thing . . . I need to feel there is some over-arching meaning to life, [otherwise] I would want to destroy it.*

For other men, the situation was a little different. Their life did have a sense of meaning, but one which was becoming eroded as they began to question it. Many men had been brought up to see pursuit of the remedies as their main goal in life. It was not necessarily that some were unsuccessful in attaining these goals, but that the goals themselves were becoming critiqued and found wanting; a sense of '*Is this it?*' William above described a creeping disillusionment with these goals; others linked their questioning to a specific event. In particular, questioning was often prompted by what the existentialist philosopher Jaspers (1986) called a limit situation, an experience which forces one to confront mortality. In the narratives, this was often the illness and/or death of a loved one. Such bereavement experiences can destabilise the foundations of a person's existence, compelling a re-evaluation of priorities, a yearning for new meaning to make sense of the tragedy (Neimeyer, 2006). Grant's early adulthood had been characterised by materialism, and the pursuit of money and success. The death of his partner made him reconsider the importance of his well-remunerated career.

> *There was this terrible sense of sadness . . . and then this, 'I've got to do something with my life, more than just being rich.' I realised I was incredibly lucky to be alive . . . It taught me the value of human life . . . a sort of, 'Phew, make the most of it.'*

As dissatisfaction prompted questioning and re-evaluation of their way of being, men began to look around for alternatives. This desire for meaning, or at least curiosity to explore other ways of living, prompted a period of searching, the archetypal existential 'quest' for meaning (Wong & Fry, 1998). For some, their seeking took them abroad. Again, Asia was a common destination, which perhaps reflects a long-standing notion within Western societies around the 'mystery' of the East, a trope which Said (1995) described pejoratively as 'orientalism'. However, there are clear differences between these seekers and those who found meditation through the two reasons outlined above. In contrast to those men who stumbled on Buddhism in Asia through a pursuit of hedonism, these men had a much more definite sense of looking for meaning, a vivid feeling that they were lacking something. In contrast to men in the first group – who had also been searching for meaning and alternative ways of being – men in this third existential questioning group exuded a much greater sense of *desperation*, of being lost in life, of *'needing a framework to cling on to'*, in Dalton's words. For men seeking in Asia, their questioning was intensified by the contrast between their unhappiness and the apparent happiness of those around. The contrast was especially perplexing given men's own greater relative prosperity, which they had been 'taught' would lead to wellbeing. As John recalled:

> *I thought, 'I can't go on like this'...People [there] seemed happier than me, and I've supposedly got all the things I want...I remember feeling very desperate, not really having a clear sense of who I was, or what I was doing. I cried and felt a bit desolate.*

While these men had not previously actively sought spiritual engagement, they had not closed themselves off to its possibility either. In this mode of seeking, they enquired into spiritual discourses and practices, like visiting monasteries on their travels. Danny was intrigued by paintings of the Buddha, and the message that *'he wasn't the son of God, and he could see there was suffering in the world, and had answers'*. In this spirit of openness, he stayed at a monastery, where he had some powerful experiences, including a moment of insight of *'love being the right way to live in the world'*. Thus, Buddhism seemed a potential gateway to a more meaningful existence. We can also appreciate why men were drawn to Buddhism *specifically*, as opposed to other systems of meaning. Some men experimented with different spiritualities before alighting on Buddhism as the one which best suited them. Some scholars describe this process of checking out different practices in pejorative terms as 'shopping' in a 'spiritual supermarket' (Redden, 2005). However, since in a globalised world one *does* have access to a whole field of alternatives, the idea of consciously choosing a spiritual orientation (rather than simply inheriting one on the basis of one's cultural location) makes sense. With men having rejected Christianity for its homophobic tendencies, or from their inability to believe in God, Buddhism offered an appealing alternative.

> *I looked carefully at Christianity, but I never believed in God... I went off for another two year trip, had a good look at Hinduism, a look at Islam, but realised quickly that Islam was definitely a no-no, and Hinduism is pretty hopeless if you're gay... I came across the Tibetans. They treated me beautifully, [and] were completely accepting... and there was no real God involved, [which] made it simpler.* (Grant)

Not all of those unhappy with their life needed to travel to encounter new possibilities. A few men, despite their dissatisfaction with life, had not actively set out on a search for meaning. While William had begun to question the remedies – *'Is this it?'* – he had not embarked on an existential quest, nor gone abroad in search of alternatives. Instead, he stumbled on a solution closer to home, meeting a Buddhist who seemed to offer an alternative to his current way of living. His narrative highlights the way issues around meaning intersect with gender. His constricted sense of the possibilities in life was tied into restrictions he felt in relation to masculinity: he had a narrow vision of how men could act in the world. While he valued non-traditional qualities (*'I'm very pro feminine-type blokes'*), he rarely met such men (*'I spent most of my life trying to work round excessively testosterone-fuelled men'*). Thus, although he felt there could be more to life than the remedies, since all the men around him were also pursuing these, he came to see these as just what men 'do'. However, he was intrigued by a sports team-mate who offered an attractive alternative masculinity (*'More feminine than a caricature of a masculine man'*). Hearing that this man was a Buddhist was portrayed as a revelation, as it seemed to suggest the possibility of exploring a different way of being a man.

> *I'd known [him] as this nice, gentle man, but just somebody who I played [sport] with and then went to the pub with... [Someone said], 'He's going*

to work at this Buddhist centre.' Everybody was, 'Wow, that's crazy', and I was, 'Yeah, that's wild.'

Although these men had identified meditation and/or Buddhism as potentially offering the sense of meaning they were looking for, taking it up was a bold move. William said attending a class was an *'unusual'* departure from the standard evening fare of either *'go to the pub, do some sport, or go home and watch TV'*. Nevertheless, these men were sufficiently curious and emboldened to resist social pressure and step out of usual patterns of behaviour. For men who had felt restricted by expectations in the past, like those with a constrictive upbringing, starting meditation was a liberating act of self-determination. John reminisced about thinking: ' "*I'm not doing this because anyone wants me to. I'm doing this because I want to*" ...*I'd made that decision, and just felt freer.'* Although these men had faced a challenging period of existential questioning, they appreciated the new possibilities for living seemingly offered by meditation/Buddhism. However, this still leaves a small number of men who did not have the tenacity to go searching for alternatives or the fortune to stumble upon them. While such men were often dissatisfied with their way of living – relying on the remedies for their wellbeing – they were unable or unwilling to countenance something different; they carried on running in the same circles until a crisis compelled them to try to change, as the next section explores.

Crisis/breakdown

Finally, about a third of men only found their way to meditation following a crisis. Such men had parallels with those who found meditation through the reasons above, but also crucial differences. Like those who began meditating in the hope of better dealing with stress, these men had trouble managing their emotions, often looking to the remedies to solve their issues (e.g., blunting their emotions with drink). Like those who found meditation after existential questioning, these men felt dissatisfied with their existence, and often yearned for a new way of living. Crucially though, *unlike* the men above, these men did not seek or find a way out of their predicament. Despite a growing failure of the remedies to provide them with wellbeing, these men could see no alternative. A key factor here was their perception of spirituality. This last group of men generally conflated religion and spirituality, and so having rejected the former, had also closed themselves off to the latter. Thus, while they were often aware of alternatives like meditation, they regarded it as too 'flaky' for the rational man they saw themselves as. For instance,

Terry viewed meditation as *'what spiritual people do, and I'm not a spiritual person'*. With contemplation of alternatives discouraged by his secular, well-educated peer group, he recalled thinking:

> *'It's all a load of rubbish, wishy-washy, hocus-pocus, airy-fairy'...I didn't talk about religion, or God or the meaning of life...They just weren't the kinds of conversations that were had with my circle of friends.*

While these men felt unhappy in life, they were unable to see a way out of their distress. They articulated a claustrophobic sense of feeling existentially 'trapped'. As Dalton said: *'I saw an endless life stretching ahead of me. It just seemed a bit pointless, the whole thing, and there didn't seem any relief.'* Here we find vivid accounts of the themes discussed at the end of the previous chapter. These were men in considerable distress; however, having previously been encouraged to disconnect from their emotions, they were at a loss how to resolve their issues. In vain these men looked to the remedies as a solution to their plight, but these ultimately proved unsuccessful in the ways outlined above. For example, men threw themselves into work, or sought to blunt their emotions with alcohol/drugs. However, there was an increasing sense of helplessness as the inadequacies of their coping strategies became apparent. Without a 'way out', these men portrayed issues escalating and intensifying, reflecting Brownhill and colleagues' (2005) concept of the 'big build', which depicts the way men often fail to address emotional issues until these reach a crisis point. Steven recalled his recurrent depression, his inability to envisage a solution, and a sense of *'desperation'*.

> *I could see these depressions getting closer and closer together...I was trapped by this mortgage, having to keep doing this job I didn't want...Pressured, getting angry, going round and round...thinking, 'I'm trapped in this forever, I'm always going to be like this.'*

Crucially, despite their escalating distress, these men still did not reach out or seek help. The narratives here corroborate studies suggesting that masculinity norms around toughness mean men are often unwilling to admit to vulnerabilities, preferring to hide their weaknesses and struggle on alone (Addis & Mahalik, 2003). Thus we find support here for Addis's (2008) frameworks linking masculinity and mental health issues. Echoing the masked depression framework (Cochran & Rabinowitz, 2000), these men generally tried to conceal their suffering from others. As Colin put it, *'I was in a pretty awful state internally, [but] I'm very able to hide my difficult states.'* Not only did men themselves feel they ought to be self-sufficient, some even expected health professionals to share this view of how men should be (Dalton: *'I imagined [the GP] going, "Get on with your life"'*). This particular excerpt gives us food for thought in terms of how men's reluctance to seek help may be exacerbated by perceptions of the healthcare system. As it was, these men battled on alone. Norms of self-sufficiency were so potent and pervasive that even men who otherwise resisted hegemonic expectations were influenced by them. For example, Silas was an emotionally articulate gay man who was guided by caring ideals into a healthcare career. Even so, he still recalled:

> *I had a view that only people who were incapable in some way had therapy, who were weak. I had a view that I was able, confident. Asking for help wasn't something I did.*

As such, unwilling to seek help, and coping strategies failing – e.g., self-medication through drugs exacerbating emotional issues – these men recalled escalating distress. Eventually a tipping point was reached: a negative event or experience was the catalyst for a crisis that brought everything *'to a head'*. These precipitating events took various forms. For Dalton, it was lashing out aggressively at a colleague: *'I stood up and grabbed him…It really shocked me…I hadn't realised how stressed I'd been, I just felt so aggressive.'* For Ali, it was when he began drinking heavily in the aftermath of his marriage ending: *'I got myself arrested for being a trouble maker, got into fights, which I've never done before, but I was full of anger.'* Jack was imprisoned for antisocial behaviour, but the real nadir came when he was placed in solitary confinement while in prison: *'That was a really intense experience. I thought I was going to lose it and go over the edge.'* For many of these men, including Ali and Dalton, the context for these crises was the break-up of a relationship. This reflects the idea above of the precariousness of men relying on relationships for their wellbeing – if/when these failed, men felt completely lost. After a break-up, Silas broke down at home. It was a *'dark moment'*.

> *Physically exhausted, emotionally frail, I was in a bad way. The end of a relationship was the catalyst for a moment of wailing…[On] the floor, crying, I felt, 'I've got to change my life, this isn't working, and I don't know what to do.'*

These crises were the culmination of men's stories of bowing to traditional pressures and learning to be emotionally tough; the end-game of men's failures to deal constructively with distress, their tendency to disconnect from emotional problems. For example, in despair after a break-up, Ernest had a gnawing sense that this nadir was the conclusion of his attempts to seek *'distractions from looking within'* through the hedonism of sex and drugs: *'It was like, "Why have I run around in my 20s not looking within? Why do I not seek ways to fill my own chaos with peace?'* In this bleak moment – *'wailing, a terrible sound'* – he came close to suicide: *'I didn't realise how bad it could hurt. I looked at my airgun and I thought, "I don't want to feel like this".'* Ernest gives a heart-rending illustration of the idea that men are liable to respond to distress with 'externalising' behaviours like suicide, which accounts for higher suicide and alcoholism rates among men (Addis, 2008). In being emotionally disconnected, issues that men had long been avoiding had become *'stored up'*. In this crisis, men portrayed their mental defences, which had until then kept these problems at bay, as breaking down. As noted above, Terry had blunted his negative feelings through marijuana. After a relationship break-up, all the problems he had tried to suppress came to the surface.

> *[The break-up] caused me a huge amount of pain ... affected me really quite strongly and adversely. I had a really big dip, you can call it a breakdown. Lots of things came to a head, stuff that had been stored up for years that I hadn't looked at or dealt with properly ... I went downhill to rock-bottom.*

These crises were pivotal turning points in men's narratives. The phrase *'wake-up call'* was common. The dire nature of their predicaments made men question the way of being that had brought them to this point. Jack's incarceration was when the *'real questioning started ... My mind was completely pre-occupied with how I got there? Why did this happen? What's going on?'* Given the severity of their distress, men realised that their usual coping strategies would be inadequate. Dalton recalled thinking: *'"I've got to do more than have a few drinks" ... I had to do something a bit more radical.'* These are the kind of points in men's stories when they realised they must change. Ali recalled: *'I was on the edge of the precipice ... The only option available to me was to continue with this, along this dark tunnel, or do something to change.'*

In constructing such crises as turning points, some even suggested these had been necessary in compelling them to find more constructive ways of managing their issues (Ross: *'You have to admit defeat, and see by this constant spinning around you're not going to get anywhere. You have to hit a wall'*). In this sense, these narratives support the concept of post-traumatic growth: 'positive psychological change experienced as a result of the struggle with highly challenging life circumstances' (Tedeschi & Calhoun, 2004, p. 1). These men felt they had turned their life around as a response to these crises (i.e., by taking up meditation). As such, these crises were generally viewed with retrospective gratitude as painful interventions which were ultimately beneficial.

> *I'd suffered most of my life ... but the suffering that came as a result of [a crisis] was my wake-up call. It was life saying, 'What are you going to do about it?' ... It's the best thing that happened to me ... It made me sit up, take notice, and do something to change.* (Dustin)

However, while these crises eventually had a positive outcome, the immediate aftermath was usually very hard. Men in crisis may have felt that change was necessary. However, such was their distress that, at the time, many did not feel change was possible. Unable to conceive of a way out of their distress, some sank into despair. Ernest's break-up *'wrenched'* him apart: *'It cast a UV light. You see how fragmented you are.'* This precipitated months of depression, recalled as *'very numb, desensitising, heavy'*. Poetically, he likened the experience to being *'at the bottom of a staircase, take one step and the leg is so heavy, it's greasy and I slip back off'*. In these depths, he felt very alone: *'There's a sheet of glass at the top. Everyone's saying it will be ok, but you can't quite hear it, it's stifled.'* In contrast to the nadir of contemplating suicide, which as an externalising behaviour reflects the idea of male-specific depression, this aftermath was closer to traditional conceptions of depression (e.g., lethargy). Until this point, men had tried to conceal their distress. However, they had reached such a low ebb that they had no choice but to finally seek help (Silas: *'I was so done in I just recognised it very plainly, "You need to do something"'*). Even then, men were still reluctant: Dustin said that starting counselling was *'the hardest decision I ever made'*. Having spent years disconnecting from his emotional issues, his resistance was linked to anxiety about what might be uncovered.

> *It took three months to make the call ... It's the fear of what might come out ... It's as if there are two states of coexistence. There's the knowledge that something's not right and you need to do something. And yet ... the fear holds you back.*

Having taken the step of seeking help, men found therapy immensely helpful. Whatever the specific concerns men took to the sessions, it was a relief simply to admit their distress. It is suggested that men often make for recalcitrant and uncommunicative clients in therapy (Meth et al., 1991). However, these men appreciated the chance to relinquish their tough stance. Just opening up to a sympathetic listener was in itself helpful. For Terry, aside from the specific therapeutic insights he went on to receive, just having another person hear and acknowledge his suffering was significant: '*What I needed, and this tells the whole story of what got me to that point, was someone that would really listen and take my distress seriously.*' Men valued therapy for allowing them to move away from the restrictive models of masculinity that since childhood had cramped their emotional life and contributed to their breakdown. For example, before his breakdown and subsequent therapy, Dalton could remember '*wanting to do away with the old rules... this idea of who I'm supposed to be*'. However, he had been unable to go '*into that area of being upset*' until he started therapy and felt he was allowed to be '*able to cry*'. In this permissive space, men were finally able to explore emotions and issues they had previously disconnected from. As Colin said: '*I needed to be angry, I needed to talk, I needed to blame, I needed to sort of figure out, "So what?"*' Similarly, Dalton recalled:

> *I started exploring... I began to look at all the issues that I'd been hiding away from, during childhood and university, being able to really say stuff to my therapist that had stayed buried for so many years. It was just such a relief really.*

Therapy enabled these men to gradually emerge from their distress, and feel more stable. We might say that therapy helped them understand the past, and also feel more comfortable in the present. Indeed, one of the central functions of psychotherapy is enabling the client to come to terms with their history in such a way that allows them to function well in their present life (Gonçalves, 1994). However, crucially, this still left the future uncertain. As therapy came to an end, men felt something else would be needed to help from then on. Dalton: '*I wanted to move forwards into something and build something in my life, particularly around values, and move towards more positivity.*' In a similar way, although Steven had seen his GP about his recurrent depression, '*the doctor's answer was always Prozac*'. While this would work for a time, Steven knew the depression '*was going to come back around again*'. As such, he eventually began to seek '*some other solution*'. In this spirit of trying to find a constructive way forward, many of these men said their therapist had recommended meditation to them. Some men were resistant, especially as these men had mostly been antipathetic to spirituality previously. However, they had sufficient trust in their therapist to try it. Silas recalled:

> *I was talking to [my therapist] about the psychotherapeutic process, and what to do next. He said, 'Why don't you try meditation?' I thought, 'Oooh that's interesting'. I hadn't even considered any kind of working on myself in that way.*

However, despite the progress men had made in therapy, they were still finding their way out of their breakdown, and many still felt fragile. Attending a meditation group meant venturing into unknown territory. Many had been wary of trying alternatives before their breakdown; in their vulnerable state, this was even more challenging. As mentioned above, meditation often contravened expectations of peer groups, society generally, and even men's families. Those men who experienced a crisis were more likely to be those who had previously had difficulty challenging gendered expectations. As such, concern about transgressing norms was a further barrier to engagement with meditation. Dalton procrastinated for a year before attending his local centre: '*[It was] stepping outside my limits. I'm quite cautious as a person, and no-body I knew meditated. I felt anxious about coming down on my own ... wary [and] scared.*' Given that these men were just finding their way out of an emotional crisis, taking the decision to try meditation was a bold step. For example, Terry recalled '*trying to work my way out of depths of depression*' in therapy. With Christmas '*looming*' he wanted to be '*around kind, gentle people*'. Having seen an advert for a retreat, he felt this would meet his needs. However, he only went after phoning the retreat leader, who assuaged his worries.

> *I was really fragile, very vulnerable, moods were so unpredictable. I thought, 'Is that actually safe? What if I don't like it? Will I be able to escape? Am I strong enough to be around a whole lot of strangers?' ... He reassured me it would be suitable ... people would look out for me ... That swung it.*

Thus, in spite of their concerns, in various ways, all participants eventually took up some form of meditation. Men's experiences of meditation are the focus of the next chapter.

Summary

In the last chapter, we saw how participants became disconnected from their inner emotional world, with deleterious consequences for their wellbeing: participants lacked the skill to deal constructively with their distress, or pursue wellbeing generally. However, it was not the case that men did not *try* to manage their wellbeing. As this chapter elucidates, men turned to four 'remedies' which they hoped would alleviate their troubles and otherwise meet their needs: romantic relationships; drink/drugs; work and achievement; and hobbies. However, these responses were 'precarious': even if they worked for a time, they were ultimately ineffectual, and even counterproductive. Finally, men turned to meditation as a solution, doing so when they realised that the remedies were not viable solutions to their problems. However, there were different reasons men found meditation: exploring other ways of being; in response to stress; following existential questioning; and after a crisis. Such reasons constituted predicaments of escalating 'seriousness'. Men who found meditation via the first route had a relatively easy journey. Those who required a crisis to compel them to try something different had a much harder route, often involving serious emotional and social issues. Nevertheless, in their various ways, all participants eventually took up a meditation practice, as the next chapter explores.

4
Turning Inwards through Meditation

It's very easy to look at meditation [as] you shut your eyes, do the pose. [But] it's about reflection, finding out where you're at, what makes you tick...going deep [and] being introspective. (Ali)

So far we have seen that, encouraged by masculinity norms around toughness, men often became disconnected from their inner world. This meant that men had trouble engaging with their emotions, and as such, found it difficult to deal with distress. Various 'remedies' men hoped would take care of their problems proved ultimately ineffectual. Thus, men eventually turned to meditation in the hope of finding a better solution to the particular burdens they were struggling under. Now, these next two chapters focus on meditation itself. This chapter describes how meditation was primarily a way for men to become more aware of their inner world. The next chapter explores the way this awareness helped men to better manage their emotions, thus engendering wellbeing.

This chapter is in two parts. The first gives a brief overview of the historical origins of meditation, with a particular focus on its Buddhist roots (since many participants practised in a Buddhist context). The second focuses on the different types of meditation practised by men here, where it will become apparent that all these types pertain in various ways to the development of attention.

The roots of meditation

In contemporary society, meditation has come to assume an almost ubiquitous presence. It is discussed widely in the media, in broadsheet (The Guardian, 2013) and tabloid newspapers (The Mirror, 2011), in science magazines (The New Scientist, 2011) and on news networks (CNN, 2012). It is used to sell everything from cars (Archive of Adverts and Commercials [AAC], 2002) and beer (AAC, 2012) to furniture (AAC, 2008) and dog food (AAC, 2007). It has been adapted for use in all manner of settings, from schools (Erricker & Erricker, 2001) and prisons (Bowen et al., 2006) to hospitals (Kabat-Zinn, 2003) and corporate workplaces (Schmidt-Wilk et al., 1996). However, there is considerable confusion as to what meditation actually is (Cardoso et al., 2004). As we shall see, meditation takes many different forms. Moreover, although meditation is frequently associated with Eastern religions, most societies have historically developed their own forms of meditative practices. Thus, this section starts by giving a brief tour of the different forms of meditation that have been devised across the world's cultures. However, since many of the men here practised within a Buddhist context, the section then introduces Buddhism in a little more detail, including the way it has become transmitted to, and adapted for, the 'West'.

To get a sense of the universality of meditation – as opposed to being narrowly thought of as an 'Eastern' practice – we begin by considering the way in which the word 'meditation' has evolved historically (Fisher, 2006). Its etymological roots are in the Latin term *meditatio*, meaning to engage in reflection. Although the term was originally used in the West to refer to all types of intellectual exercise, it began to be employed more specifically as a synonym of contemplation. Contemplation could take various objects as its focus. Within philosophy, it became common to speak of 'meditations' on particular themes, such as Descartes' (1641) 'meditation' on the nature of the human mind. Similarly, the term meditation was used within religious contexts to describe reflection on aspects of the Christian narrative. For example, we see descriptions of Christians engaged in 'ardent contemplation of the sufferings of Christ on the Cross' (Wildegren, 1961, p. 169). Thus, forms of contemplative prayer in Christianity constitute examples of meditative practices that have developed in the West (Ryan, 2001).

Indeed, most religious traditions have developed their own meditative practices. In Islam, for example, Sufism has a form of worship known as 'Sama', involving 'reverently listening to music and/or the singing of mystical poetry with the intent of increasing awareness and understanding of the divine object described' (Lewisohn, 1997, p. 3). Similarly, in Judaism we find a wealth of contemplative practices. For instance, in the Kabbalistic tradition, there are meditations where the practitioner is implored to 'attach' himself to God by visualising the letters of His 'Unique Name' as if written before them in the Torah (Ashurit script), such that each letter appears 'infinitely large' (Kaplan, 1989, p. 142). Then of course there is Hinduism, which is thought to have developed the earliest examples of meditation. (Earthenware seals dating back to 3000 BC, found in excavations of cities of the Indus Valley civilisation, depict figures seated in the traditional cross-legged meditation pose; Varenne, 1977.) In Hinduism, a comprehensive system of physical, mental and spiritual disciplines was developed. These are collectively referred to as 'yoga', a Sanskrit term derived from the verb *yug*, meaning to bind or to yoke together. Thus yoga is often interpreted as meaning to 'unite the mind and body in a way that promotes health' (Wren et al., 2011, p. 477).

The forms of meditation practised by men here derived mainly from Buddhism, a tradition built on the teachings of Siddhartha Gautama. The historical existence of Gautama – better known by the honorific *Buddha*, meaning 'Enlightened one' – is undisputed (Harvey, 1990). Although Indological scholars have been unable to ascertain his precise biographical dates, there is some preference for believing that he was born around 480 BC and died around 400 BC (Cousins, 1996). His birthplace is similarly contested (Thomas, 2000); however, after the discovery in 1895 of a pillar erected by the Indian Emperor Ashoka in 249 BC near Lumbini (in the central Tarai plain of present day Nepal), in 1997 UNESCO awarded World Heritage Status to the site as his official birthplace (UNESCO, 1997). The cultural context of his time was one in which the Hindu religion dominated, which promoted yoga practices that would later come to be adapted by Gautama as he developed his own teachings and system of meditation (Dumoulin, 1979). Reliable accounts of the historical development of Buddhism are hampered by the lack of historicity of the source documents; i.e., they were not written to provide a factual account as we would understand it, but rather to mythologise the life of its founder (Harvey, 1990). In this vein, Gautama's life is usually articulated with the following narrative (Gyatso, 2007).

Gautama is believed to have been raised in relative luxury as the son of the chief of the Sakya clan. He lived a sheltered existence until age 29, when a series of encounters with people who were ill or dying prompted an existential crisis, compelling him to leave his young family and pursue a religious existence dedicated to exploring the 'human condition' (Kumar, 2002). He spent five years engaging in austere yogic practices among a company of ascetics. However, he determined that such self-mortification was unhelpful and so decided to pursue a 'middle path', i.e., between indulgence and asceticism. The legend has it that he resolved to meditate until he gained enlightenment, and sat under a pipal tree in Bodh Gaya for 49 days until, aged 35, enlightenment was attained. He spent the next 45 years formulating and propagating his insights, which are known by the Sanskrit term '*Dharma*', which carries connotations of 'laws', or 'how things are' (Kabat-Zinn, 2003). Central to the teachings are the 'Four Noble Truths', a remedy in the form of a medical diagnosis for the alleviation of suffering: suffering is universal; it has a cause; cessation is possible; achieved by following the 'Noble Eight-fold Path'. The path is a prescription for 'right living', which includes meditation and other moral recommendations – right vision, conception, speech, conduct, livelihood, effort, mindfulness and concentration (Thrangu, 1993).

Since the Buddha's death, Buddhism has developed along multiple lines as various traditions have interpreted his teachings in different ways. The early Theravadan tradition – called the 'lesser vehicle', but which literally means ancient or primordial – emerged about 100 years after the Buddha's death, and adheres rigidly to the original scriptures. The later Mahayana tradition ('greater vehicle'), which came into being around 0 AD, was more innovative and developed sophisticated philosophies by extending the original teachings (Harvey, 1990). Mahayana itself produced other traditions, including Zen – a Japanese word derived from the mandarin Chinese '*Chan*' – which resulted from Buddhism being transmitted into China around the 6th century AD. Influenced by indigenous Chinese schools of thought, namely Taoism and Confucianism, Zen developed as a less mythological and more direct Buddhism. Since then, Buddhist ideas and practices have continued to migrate and consequently evolve as they have been carried to new audiences around the world. As when Buddhism mingled with Chinese thought and took on a particular inflection in the form of Zen, Buddhism has often been adapted to suit the social and intellectual climate of these new terrains. This has been the case as Buddhism has begun to move 'Westwards'.

Buddhism was known to the West as early as the 13th century through the accounts of Marco Polo (Abeydeera, 2000). However, it was only in the late 19th century that it started becoming a cultural force as translations of scriptures became more available and religious figures from Asia began to travel abroad, e.g., attending the 1893 World Fair in Chicago. It then reached a wider audience still in the mid-20th century through influential proponents like Carl Jung, and phenomena like the 'Beat' movement (Baumann & Prebish, 2000). In this process of cultural transmission, various forms of Buddhism have been brought to the West. As suggested in the last chapter, this accessibility to a panoply of cultural practices from all around the globe has been called a spiritual supermarket (Redden, 2005). Indeed, contemporary seekers in the UK can sample a diverse variety of Buddhist forms, including Theravadan, Mahayanan and Zen traditions (Buddhanet, 2013). However, while evidently influenced by these antecedent traditions, these forms are seen as having subtly evolved to accommodate themselves to their new Western audiences. Thus, these emergent Buddhist groups in the West, even if they locate themselves within antecedent Eastern traditions, are seen by religious scholars as 'new religious movements' (NRMs) (Dawson, 1998).

As an example of the way new forms of Buddhism have evolved in Western settings, we can consider the specific movement to which a number of men here were aligned. This movement is generally known as the Friends of the Western Buddhist Order (FWBO; encompassing the more exclusive 'Western Buddhist Order', which comprises only ordained practitioners). The FWBO was founded by Dennis Lingwood, born in London in 1925. Lingwood was posted to India during World War II, and stayed on to pursue an interest in Buddhism. Whilst there, he studied under various Buddhist masters, including Dhardo Rimpoche, the teacher of the Dalai Lama. He was ordained as a Buddhist monastic in 1950, and received an honorific 'dharma name' – bestowed upon monks in the Theravadan tradition in which he practised – namely, Urgyen Sangharakshita, a Pali term meaning 'Protector of the Sangha [community]'. He remained in India until 1964, when he returned to England. After two years leading the English Sangha Trust, he founded the FWBO in 1967 (Sangharakshita, 1997). Although no longer taking an active role in leading the movement, he remains its figurehead (Vajragupta, 2010). Today, the movement is one of the largest in the UK, with over 80 affiliated groups (Bluck, 2006).

The FWBO promotes two primary meditation practices: the mindfulness of breathing and the *metta bhavana* (translated as a 'practice of loving kindness'). In addition, there are advanced practices intended for experienced meditators, like the 'Six element' practice. These will all be discussed in detail below. What is interesting in the context of the notion of NRMs is the way Sangharakshita is seen by other Buddhists as creating a new order *ex nihilo* (Vishvapani, 2001). The key practices derive from Theravadan Buddhism. However, Sangharakshita also included practical and doctrinal elements from other traditions, including Mahayanan rituals and Tibetan mantras. Subhuti (1994) describes this selectivity as an attempt to offer a 'core of common material' constituting the 'essence' of Buddhism which, divested of anachronistic cultural accretions, is 'relevant' to the West. However, his selectivity has put the FWBO at odds with traditionalists who value the 'authority of lineage and Asian precedent' (Vishvapani, 2001). (Interestingly, the FWBO was renamed in 2010 as the Triratna Buddhist Order/Community, eschewing the word 'Western' to reflect the dissemination and migration of the movement across the world. This highlights the complexities of the flow of cultural practices in our globalised age, since although the FWBO was created as a 'Western' form of Buddhism, India currently has the most FWBO members.)

The FWBO also has other features that further distinguish it from traditional Buddhist forms (Chryssides & Wilkins, 2006). First, it is neither lay nor monastic, but has three grades of involvement. *Friends* are those who practise in the movement, but not necessarily with any explicit or exclusive commitment. *Mitras* are people who have avowed, in a public ceremony, to explore Buddhism within the context of the FWBO. *Ordinants* have 'pledged themselves to follow the Buddhist path of enlightenment' (The Buddhist Centre, 2013, para. 2). A second distinguishing feature is that most of its centres are located in inner-city environments, often in impoverished areas. For example, the FWBO's largest centre is in Bethnal Green, East London, which falls in the 'most deprived' band on seven of the eight ONS (2011a) indices of deprivation. A third distinctive feature is an ethos of gender equality, which is relatively unusual in Buddhism: despite declarations from the Buddha about the 'spiritual potential' of women (Schak, 2008), Faure (2003, p. 9) argues that 'like most clerical discourses' Buddhism is 'relentlessly misogynistic'. That said, while the movement has avowedly sought to develop only a 'minimal institutional structure...of power' (Hayes, 1995, p. 6), gender ratios in the FWBO mean that men still hold positions of authority (Lokhabandhu, 2007).

I will explore participants' engagement with Buddhism in the next chapter. There we will see that meditation was part of a broader framework of ideas and practices that many men found conducive to wellbeing, like a sense of community. As such, when considering the meditation practices in the section below, it is important to appreciate that, for most men, these were generally set within this larger Buddhist context. This is relevant, as much of the scientific literature on meditation presents it in a decontextualised way, where its Buddhist/Hindu roots are not explicitly acknowledged (Shapiro, 1994). For example, there has recently been much clinical interest in mindfulness (see below). However, this has generally become dissociated from its Theravadan roots and co-opted into a Western medical framework.

This particular adaptation of Buddhism has been labelled 'scientific Buddhism' (McMahan, 2004). That is, paradoxically, one way in which Buddhism has been tailored for Western audiences has been to divest it of the religious connotations of Buddhism itself, and present it in secular terms as a medical-therapeutic practice (Obadia, 2008). However, as noted in the last chapter, one of the reasons men were drawn to try meditation was because they were particularly intrigued by Buddhism. For example, Dean recalled:

> *I had a vague idea [that Buddhism] was about wisdom and compassion and some things being more important than money. The Dalai Lama embodies that, the Tibetan equivalent to Nelson Mandela...something about peace and wisdom.*

Thus, as we look at the different types of meditation that participants practised, it is worth bearing in mind this larger context. Meditation was not an isolated activity, detached from a cultural location – it sat within a broader network of people, places and practices influenced by Buddhism. For example, as we read about men's experiences of trying to meditate below, we should remember that these are not descriptions of a disembodied process, but involved real men in actual social situations. For example, for many men, the first time they meditated was in a Buddhist centre. In considering their depictions of the experience, it helps to recall that these were men who had been taught that it is important to be tough, who had struggled to connect with their emotions, who tried to ignore or repress their distress, who had often faced a painful route to reach the point where they would even consider meditation, who even then had to overcome social pressures that discouraged them from attending. In this context, we can that appreciate it was a big step for many to even sit down to meditate in the first place. Dalton recalled his worries about going to the Buddhist centre for the first time.

> *No-body I knew meditated, so I couldn't kind of go along with anyone I knew, all my mates just wanted to go down the pub and drink...I felt anxious about coming down on my own...I didn't know much about Buddhism but I imagined that it would be full of Tibetan monks or something...But it was so local that I thought, 'Ok, I'll go there.' So eventually, stressed, I pushed myself to go down.*

Types of meditation

Across men's narratives – and throughout Buddhism generally – there are a diverse array of meditation practices. To help make sense of these various forms, we can differentiate these according to four parameters (Mikulas, 1990): behaviours of mind; object; attitude; and form. As will become apparent, these parameters all pertain to the deployment of *attention*. Thus, first and foremost, meditation is about learning to pay attention: this is its defining characteristic. As Goleman (1988, p. 107) says, 'the need for the meditator to retrain his attention . . . is the single invariant ingredient . . . of every meditation system'. So, taking the four parameters in turn: 'behaviours of mind' refers to the *types* of attention that meditation practices can involve; 'object' concerns the different stimuli that can be the *focus* of attention in meditation; 'attitude' is the *emotional quality* with which meditators are encouraged to suffuse their attention; and 'form' relates to different *physical postures* that can be adopted in meditation to encourage the deployment of attention. This section considers these different parameters in turn, using them to show the range of practices that men here engaged in, but also to emphasise that these practices all essentially involved the development of attention.

Types of attention

Above all else, contemporary theorists see meditation as a system for training attention. This is not necessarily the way meditation has been conceptualised classically within the religious traditions that first developed the various meditation practices. The concept of attention is a modern construct produced by a system of thought that, influenced by computer metaphors, views the mind in rather mechanistic terms (Crowther-Heyck, 1999). In contrast, religious traditions were given to presenting meditation using more poetic discourses. That said, these early depictions are close enough to contemporary psychological thought that their translation into modern scientific terms is not untenable. For example, in a *sutra* (aphorism) attributed to the Buddha, instructions for a meditation on the sun begin as follows: '[C]ause your mind to be firmly fixed on it so as to have an unwavering perception by the exclusive application of your mind' (Buddha, 1894, part II, verse 9). From this excerpt we can see that approaching meditation with the conceptual tools of modern psychology is not necessarily *too* far removed from the ideas that we can discern within the original passages.

Thus, we find that theorists today have primarily honed in on the concept of attention as the defining feature of meditation. Across the myriad different forms of practice, learning how to skilfully deploy attention is viewed as the common denominator. As Cahn and Polich (2006, p. 180) put it, 'regulation of attention is the central commonality across the many divergent methods'. Similarly, Walsh and Shapiro (2006, pp. 228–229) define meditation generally as 'a family of self-regulation practices that focus on training attention and awareness in order to bring mental processes under greater voluntary control and thereby foster general mental well-being'. As this quote indicates, sometimes scholars speak of attention and awareness – often using these rather interchangeably (although as will be set out below, these are distinct concepts). Indeed, most participants here tended to speak about meditation as fundamentally about developing awareness, rather than using the more psychological concept of attention. For example, Walter described meditation as '*a tool that basically refines my awareness ... a practice of building awareness*'. Andrew drew on both concepts – awareness and attention – in articulating his own definition of meditation.

> *It's about expanding your awareness out to check what your mind is doing. Other-wise it's like you're trying to drive with the handbrake on, [not] paying attention ... to the smell coming from the wheels ... Now I can hear the wheels, and smell the burning rubber. This checking attitude is about [asking], 'How does my mind feel right now?' Nothing complicated about it, just 'What's the state of my mind at the moment?'*

Thus, we can depict meditation as involving the development of attention *and/or* awareness. Importantly, the reason that Mikulas (1990) presented 'behaviours of mind' as a *parameter* is that meditation practices can utilise and invoke different *types* of attention and awareness. Thus, before we consider the different types of practices, it is worth clarifying what we mean by attention and awareness, since though they are often used synonymously, they are distinct concepts (Koch & Tsuchiya, 2007). Essentially, awareness is conscious experience, whereas attention refers to the cognitive mechanisms that control what *enters* awareness. Moreover, we can be even more specific, and identify different types of both awareness and attention.

Awareness is subdivided into 'phenomenal' and 'access' awareness. Phenomenal awareness refers to subjectivity, a catch-all term for the experience of qualia, i.e., the sensation of 'what it is like to be' a particular person enjoying a particular experience (Nagel, 1974). Access awareness refers to the more limited case of subjective experience being available for 'use in reasoning and rationally guiding speech and action' (Block, 1995, p. 227). Phenomenal awareness itself comprises subtypes pertaining to different sensory modalities, such as visual awareness, as well as other information sources including interoceptive (body sensations) and proprioceptive awareness (body movement) (Sarrazin et al., 2008). There are also higher forms of reflexive meta-awareness of one's mental processes, e.g., of thoughts (Siegel, 2007). Awareness *without* content may even be possible, involving just a bare 'field' of awareness (Josipovic, 2010). This is referred to as 'non-dual' awareness, since it involves the dissipation of the dualistic subject–object construct, i.e., a subject who is aware of an object (Travis & Shear, 2010). While non-dual awareness is a disputed phenomenon, and may be rarely achieved in practice, it is linked by scholars to advanced meditation skills.

In contrast, attention refers to mechanisms which control what enters awareness (Fell, 2004). This involves enhancement of the way information is processed from a particular area of the sensory field: attention modulates cognitive and perceptual processing by directing resources to relevant internal or external stimuli (Rafal & Posner, 1987). As Austin (1998, p. 69; italics in original) puts it, while awareness involves sensate 'reactivity', attention is a 'searchlight': 'Attention reaches. It is awareness stretched *toward* something. It has executive, motoric implications. We attend *to* things.' Attention is theorised as being modular, comprising three functionally distinct but overlapping networks (Posner & Petersen, 1990). Sustained attention concerns the intensity of attention, and refers to on-going readiness for processing stimuli, involving extended mental effort over time (Hilti et al., 2010). The other networks concern attentional selectivity: executive attention is the top-down monitoring of competing stimuli; selective attention is when resources are allocated to specific stimuli (Müller & Rabbitt, 1989). In addition, Mirsky and colleagues (1991, p. 112) identified attention switching as 'the ability to change attentive focus in an adaptable and flexible manner'.

With meditation, contemporary theorists classify practices into two types: focused attention (FA) and open monitoring (OM) (Lutz et al., 2008). Buddhism uses 'Pali', the Indian language of early Buddhist texts, to refer to these respectively as '*samatha*' and '*vipassana*'. FA practices primarily involve sustained attention, focusing on a particular object such as the breath; however, they also utilise the other attention networks: monitoring (to prevent the mind 'wandering'), switching (disengaging from distractions), and selective (redirecting focus back to the meditative object). In contrast, OM does not involve focusing attention on particular stimuli, but rather describes a broad receptive awareness. As Raffone and Srinivasan (2010, p. 2) explain it, OM is 'an open field capacity to detect arising sensory, feeling and thought events within an unrestricted "background" of awareness, without a grasping of these events in an explicitly selected foreground or focus'. As practitioners turn inwards and introspect, thoughts, feelings and sensations are registered as they arise, without the practitioner 'clinging' to these. OM is characterised by qualities including receptivity, clarity, stability/continuity, flexibility and non-conceptual awareness, i.e., without discursive elaboration (Brown et al., 2007).

The idea of OM is often better known by the term 'mindfulness'. Mindfulness is rooted in the Theravadan practice of Vipassana (Hart, 1987), and is defined as 'the awareness that arises through paying attention on purpose, in the present moment, and nonjudgementally to the unfolding of experience moment by moment' (Kabat-Zinn, 2003, p. 145). The term is derived from the Pali word '*Sati*', which carries connotations of being watchful and alert (Kiyota, 1978). Over recent decades, mindfulness has become the pre-eminent focus of clinicians and researchers interested in meditation, generating a proliferation of 'mindfulness meditation practices' (Baer, 2003). This interest stems mainly from a Mindfulness-Based Stress Reduction (MBSR) programme founded by Kabat-Zinn (1982). Utilising ideas and practices from the Vipassana tradition, he developed an intervention that had significant success in treating patients with chronic pain. Such has been the appeal – and adaptability – of this idea of mindfulness, that it is the most widely researched and practised form of meditation in the West today (Brown et al., 2007). Indeed, mindfulness is one of the two main practices promoted by the FWBO. Thus, participants here tended to use the words 'mindfulness' and 'awareness' interchangeably – to be mindful *is* to be aware.

> *When I say mindful, I mean . . . being aware of the moment, how I'm feeling, aware of everything around me . . . What you discover is, as long as you're being mindful and in the moment whilst meditating, that's the key. You're not attempting to be anything or fight anything off. Just allow thoughts to happen and pass, give space and don't be restrictive.* (Vincent)

Although scholars have found it helpful to conceptually differentiate FA and OM, in practice, many meditation practices involve a mixture of both. It is often recommended to practitioners that they begin a practice using FA to help first calm the mind, thus preventing it 'wandering' in a more expansive phase of OM later in the practice (Lutz et al., 2008). This was confirmed in narratives here. For example, most men had tried to practise mindfulness. However, many made a point of emphasising how *difficult* it was to be mindful. As explored above, men had previously been encouraged to disconnect from their interior world. Thus turning inwards and trying to introspect was a radical step. Initially, even just sitting still was often unusual (Steven: *'I'd never done anything like sitting doing nothing for 20 minutes'*). In their first attempts of trying to practise mindfulness, men recalled an inability to concentrate on inner experience without getting distracted. Moreover, although most narratives had a development arc – men felt they had improved their meditation skills over time – many men had on-going struggles with mindfulness.

> *Meditation is never easy...I almost feel, 'Why am I doing this? I'm rubbish at it, I just can't concentrate, there's too much going on in my head.'* (William)

In explaining the difficulties involved in being mindful, participants described the subtleties of awareness. They differentiated between being conscious of something, and being mindful of it. While they were conscious during meditation, experiencing thoughts/feelings, they did not always manage to be *mindful* of those internal events. Rather than just 'having' a thought, mindfulness was described by men as *'stepping back'* and *'observing'* these with a degree of detachment. In the meditation literature, this detachment is described as 'decentring', i.e., 'the ability to observe one's thoughts and feelings as temporary, objective events in the mind, as opposed to reflections of the self that are necessarily true' (Fresco et al., 2007, p. 234). However, mindfulness was portrayed as an elusive, fragile state, capable of easily being lost, described by Peter as the mind *'wandering off'*. He said it was possible to then become aware that the mind had 'wandered off' as such, and that by *'bringing it back'*, he could regain the desired state of mindfulness. In this way, men described 'training' awareness, so they could maintain states of mindfulness for longer periods of time.

> *When I'm meditating, I can drift away, get carried away by my thoughts, but it's just training, everyone needs to train. Meditation is about building awareness.* (Walter)

In light of such difficulties in becoming mindful, in procedural terms, men said they usually began meditation sittings with a more concentrative meditative exercise, such as focusing on the breath to *'build up awareness'* (Adam). Doing this helped prevent the mind wandering off in the more open and receptive phase of mindfulness. Steven explained: *'I'm struggling with distractions as usual! [But] breathing is a way of dealing with the distractions by teaching you to concentrate.'* This initial phase of focusing on the breath is called the 'mindfulness of breathing'. (This name is misleading: rather than being an example of the expansive OM that characterises mindfulness proper, it is actually a FA practice.) However, once men's attention had been 'stabilised' by focusing on the breath, they were better able to relax into a state of genuine OM, just sitting and 'watching' their mind. In so doing, men began to explore their inner world. Meditation was an *'inner pathway'* (Ross), enabling *'inner discovery'* (Bill) of the *'inner dimension'* (Dustin), helping access an *'inner place'* (Walter), observe *'innermost feelings and thoughts'* (Grant), and develop the *'inner self'* (Alvin). Given men's previous disengagement with their inner world, turning inwards was new and very significant. Men described learning to introspect, as if for the first time.

> *Meditation is more than about calming my mind. It's more about my mind deepening, going deeper in, trying to get more in touch with my innermost feelings and thoughts.* (Grant)

Having established that there are different types of attention and awareness, we can now turn to the second parameter introduced by Mikulas (1990): the 'object' of meditation. That is, here we ask, what did men in meditation focus their attention/awareness *on* specifically?

The focus of attention/awareness

In terms of *object*, meditation can focus on a diverse range of phenomena. This focus is often directed inwardly, towards sensations, feelings and thoughts, although it can also be directed outwardly to external stimuli. Here we will consider 'inward' stimuli first. Of such internal qualia, men indicated that it was easiest to focus on visceral sensations, as these generally were less challenging than thoughts or feelings. I have already mentioned that men here were often taught, especially as beginners, to focus on the sensation of breathing. This often had the effect of stabilising attention, but could also be harnessed as a relaxation technique. For example, Danny liked to augment this focus with a visualisation exercise, imagining himself on a seashore, with the rhythm of his breath like *'the waves coming in and out'*. Another popular technique was the 'body scan', in which men would lie on the floor and direct their attention systematically to different parts of the body in turn, beginning with their toes and moving in increments up to the head. As Ditto and colleagues (2006) found, men experienced this as a relaxing process. More interesting, given men's previous disconnection from their inner world, was the way this gave men a sense of exploring uncharted internal terrain.

> *People don't have a vocabulary for their inner experience, [but] I'm trying to collate words to different subtle physical states. You get physical sensation and you give it a name ... The body has these amazing reactions ... The gradations of feeling, of pleasure, of subtlety ... That's been part of my own work over the years.* (Robert)

Men also tried to cultivate awareness of their emotions (although it is misleading to separate these from sensations – as Robert's quote indicates, sensations and emotions shaded into one another, and emotional feelings were viscerally *felt* in the body). In light of men's previous tendencies to disconnect from their emotions, there was a learning curve here. For example, Dalton felt he had received *'quite a bit of conditioning'* to not acknowledge or recognise his emotional states. As such, men described trying to pay more attention to their emotions as like a training regime. For instance, some became better acquainted with their emotions by deliberately and consciously naming these as they arose in conscious experience. Men even did this with negative emotions, in marked contrast to previous tendencies to disconnect from such emotions. Danny: *'There's quite a strong habit to not want to face difficult feelings, [but] I've just been saying, "It's just fear." I can sense that it's uncomfortable, but it's only fear. [I] just try ... to be reassuring to myself internally, and keep it in perspective.'* This process of naming emotions is a key technique in emotion-focused therapy, which aims to promote emotional management skills (Greenberg, 2004). Indeed, the next chapter explores how men's efforts to attend to emotions in meditation did help them develop such skills.

> *Every time something occurred, I would be going, 'suffering, suffering, mindfulness, mindfulness, dislike, like', literally trying to find out, 'What's going on here?' It was the beginning of understanding that emotions are not permanent, and that you can have that sort of insight into your own emotions, instead of just headlessly being this emotional animal that's blown by the wind.* (Vincent)

Thus, having stabilised their attention with FA techniques focusing on the breath, men were able to enter a more mindful OM state and 'observe' their flux of emotions. However, one reason participants had previously disconnected from their inner world was in response to experiencing difficult emotions. So, with mindfulness likened to *'turning a light on'* (Walter), as men began to *re*-connect, troubling contents were often revealed. For example, Henry was *'confronted'* with *'painful feelings'* relating to a childhood trauma that he had suppressed for years: *'[I realised] the depth of the pain that is buried. It can be very scary to know there's that very strong thing in there.'* Thus, meditation was not always a positive experience. Men eventually learned mental skills to help them manage the negative contents they encountered in meditation, as shown in the next chapter. However, even as men became more proficient at meditating, most continually faced difficult thoughts/feelings. Men stressed that meditation was not an anaesthetising relaxation technique, or *'a pill to make me feel good'* (Dalton), but was *'hard work'* (Andrew). Michael said it *'confronts you with yourself'*. When asked if he found that painful, he replied, *'I've found me painful.'* As Andrew said:

> It can be difficult... You're coming face to face with your own heart and mind... fear, anger, hatred, confusion, frustration and anxiety, all the difficult emotions. That's the whole point... everything is included.

Men faced similar troubling surprises as they learned to become mindful of their thoughts.

First, men recalled being surprised by how busy and full their minds seemed. Moreover, they were disturbed to observe how little control they appeared to have over the thinking process (William: *'I had no control over what my conscious mind was doing'*). Men had previously assumed that they existed as a free agent, in charge of their thoughts. Observing that this was not necessarily the case could be troubling. As Andrew recalled: *'There's the shock of really encountering your mind for the first time! The thought process happens independent of you. You just think incessant crazy thoughts.'* More disturbingly, many men were forcibly struck by the negative quality of their thoughts. Dean described meditation as like *'opening a can of worms'*. Walter recalled thinking *'my mind is horrible'*. Danny found *'more dark stuff than you can imagine'*. These are striking findings: most clinical literature on meditation presents it in enthusiastic terms as an unqualified good (Dobkin et al., 2012). As such, a 'striking limitation' of the work in this area is an 'absence of research on potentially harmful or negative effects' (Irving et al., 2009, p. 65). Participants here encountered negative thoughts that they were unaware they even harboured, which challenged the views they held about themselves. A few disliked the person they found within.

> *As awareness developed, I started to see things ... feelings, emotions, sensations, thoughts, loomed larger. And actually, it was a bit of a shock. I had this view of myself as helpful, but [I found] that I entertain also these thoughts of violence, or irritability, or unkindness, or lack of concern.* (Silas)

The possibility that mindfulness could uncover negative content means that the attitude with which practitioners were mindful – the third parameter – was vital. Before turning our focus to this below, it remains to mention other phenomena that could be the target of attention in meditation. Mindfulness was practised by beginners and more experienced meditators alike. However, there were more intricate practices only undertaken by practitioners deemed more 'advanced', i.e., more skilled at deploying attention. One such was the Six element practice, which the FWBO taught only to ordinants. This practice is designed to 'deconstruct' the self, referred to in Buddhist terminology as attaining 'spiritual death'. (Note: this is not a nihilistic ideology; it means the death of a narrow, constricting self-identity, and a 're-birth' into a more expansive identity; Kramer, 1988.) The practice is based on the Buddhist theory of identity, which holds that our sense of being a coherent, unified self is a cognitive illusion, a mental concept built upon an ever-changing phenomenal stream of qualia (Siderits, 2003). This philosophy of the self had been adopted by many of the more experienced participants here.

> *As a Buddhist, my belief system is that I don't have a sense of self as a singularity ... Human beings have to believe that they're solid and robust, otherwise they [go] mad, [but] then we suddenly have to shed all that. It's terrifying to think that that which we believe we are doesn't exist.* (Harry)

Thus, the object of attention in the Six element practice is this phenomenal stream of qualia. Practitioners are encouraged to focus on the way their being is dynamically constructed from six 'elements': earth (i.e., hardness/solidity, e.g., the teeth); water (i.e., viscosity/fluidity, e.g., blood); fire (i.e., temperature, e.g., sensations of hot/cold); air (i.e., motion/mobility, e.g., the breath); space (i.e., cavities, e.g., the mouth); and consciousness (i.e., subjectivity, e.g., one's thoughts/feelings) (Nhat-Tu, 2013). This practice could be very unsettling – John suggested that

Buddhism was in a *'very kindly way'* trying to challenge one's sense of self. Others found it a liberating experience. Some described the practice as a reflection on death. Sam emphasised it was not a morbid exercise, but had the paradoxical effect of helping him feel *'completely alive'*. He referenced a Buddhist notion that death is only frightening because people cling to the idea of an independently existing self which can be 'lost' (Dalton: *'Fear is only related to the fact that we think we're separate selves'*). Sam recalled a vivid experience in Asia while he was immersing himself in the practice, sparked by the strange sight of ducks drinking from a stream of blood, which challenged his concept of an animal (*'[Its] definition exploded in my brain'*). He then found this sudden conceptual re-evaluation turned reflexively upon himself. He recalled his fear of death lifting.

> *I thought, 'If it doesn't have a fixed identity, is this the case [for me]?' It set off a chain reaction, made me reflect on who I am. It shook my worldview and everything.*

> *For a few days all my fear to die had lifted ... Nothing exists as a thing and then dies and disappears, just constantly a stream of change, one thing moves into another ... I was a changed person, I've never been able to think about things in the same way.*

Thus, we can see that some types of meditative contemplation can be radically challenging. However, these also have the potential to be destabilising. In conducting a critical appraisal of meditation, it is important to be alert to potential risks associated with it. Although there has been very little academic focus on such risks, a few studies have indicated that meditation can potentially have a detrimental impact on mental health. Shapiro (1992) found that 55 per cent of a sample of meditators reported adverse psychological effects linked to meditation, including depression and/or anxiety. Other studies have found that meditation can precipitate psychosis in those with a history of the condition (Lustyk et al., 2009). Six men in my study reported that meditation had adversely affected them at times, with three describing episodes of psychosis. These issues will be dealt with more fully in the next chapter, but it is pertinent here that one man suffered a significant adverse reaction to the Six element practice. Adam had a frightening experience when he tried it, unadvised, alone as a beginner (showing why it is regarded as a more advanced practice). He emphasised that when he later learned to do it *'correctly'*, he had a *'liberating and glorious experience'* and felt '*totally open and part of life*'. However, without guidance, he had a sense of '*meaninglessness*'.

> *I crashed, I ended up lying on the floor sobbing, because I had a really strong sense of impermanence without the context, without the positivity. The crushing experience of despair was very strong... You just feel like you don't exist, you're just nothing, there's nothing really there. It's nihilistic, pretty terrifying.*

Another class of advanced practices involves deliberate FA concentration on a pre-specified mental object (in contrast to practitioners simply being mindful of whatever thoughts/feelings happen to arise). For example, Transcendental Meditation (TM) is a technique, derived from Indian Vedic psychology, that became popular in the 1970s in the West through the teachings of Maharishi Mahesh Yogi (Alexander et al., 1991). In TM, practitioners focus on a 'mantra', a personalised phrase repeated silently. In the FWBO, ordinants receive a personalised Sadhana practice, involving contemplation of a specific Buddhist figure. This practice derives from Tibetan Buddhism, which developed a complex mythology involving a pantheon of deities. Without delving into abstruse theological speculations on the ontological nature of these deities, a modern interpretation views these as representing 'components' of the Buddha's personality, or 'states of mind' encouraged by Buddhism (Cohen, 2010). For example, the deity Tara is regarded as an embodiment of compassion. Michael depicted the Sadhana as an imaginative '*drama*' where you visualise and '*meet*' the figure. Those who had been given this practice portrayed it as full of deep meaning and significance, and most were reluctant to discuss it in detail, as it was very personal. However, they hinted that it was a process where something mysterious happens. Adam called it a '*beautiful poignant time*'.

> *There's a landscape, which initially you build up, but after you've been doing it a while, it's more you just let it unfold. [Mine] is a beautiful seascape at sunset. [I] visualise the figure... sitting on a lotus.*

Thus, meditation can take a range of mental stimuli as the focus of attention, from feelings and thoughts to meaningful words or images. However, meditation does not necessarily only involve turning attention *inwards*. The Dalai Lama defines meditation in broad terms as 'a deliberate mental activity that involves cultivating familiarity, be it with a chosen object, a fact, a theme, a habit, an outlook or a way of being'

(Gyatso, 2006, p. 98). Thus focus can also be directed *outwardly* to phenomena in the external world. For example, religious worship can often centre on a shrine, involving combinations of evocative stimuli and iconography. For instance, in Tibetan Buddhism it is common to meditate upon mandalas, i.e., ornate geometric patterns laden with religious symbolism (Saso, 1990). Shrines may also contain pictures or statues of the Buddha, and other mythological figures in the Buddhist pantheon (Vessantara, 2002). In addition, a contemplative environment can be augmented through stimuli geared to appeal to other senses, whether aural (e.g., bells, chanting) or olfactory (e.g., incense). Many men here felt shrines could be powerful objects of contemplation, particularly if focused on as part of a religious ritual. This is explored in the next section, which addresses the importance of attitude.

The attitude of attention/awareness

The third parameter with which we can differentiate among meditation practices is attitude. In meditation, practitioners are not simply encouraged to become more attentive/aware; they are implored to suffuse their attention/awareness with particular attitudinal *qualities*. For example, Kabat-Zinn's (2003) definition of mindfulness is 'awareness that arises through paying attention on purpose, in the present moment, and *nonjudgementally* to the unfolding of experience moment by moment' (p. 145; my italics). Kabat-Zinn also suggests mindfulness should ideally be conducted with an 'open-hearted, friendly' and 'affectionate, compassionate quality'. More ominously, Shapiro and colleagues (2006, p. 376) advise that mindfulness be practised in a 'compassionate' spirit, otherwise attention has the potential to 'have a cold, critical quality'. However, the writers do not draw out the negative implication of this; i.e., if one is unable to do this, meditation has the potential to be an exercise in self-criticism. This was the case here. Silas depicted awareness as '*a sledgehammer*' that he was prone to using for '*harsh, critical analysis*' of himself. Given the negativity some men encountered within, plus their tendencies towards self-criticism and low self-esteem, mindfulness could leave men feeling bad about themselves.

> *You become aware that perhaps you don't like yourself sometimes ... You just become aware, 'Actually, I'm a bit of a shit really and I'm really rude to people.' If you've got a tendency towards negativity, [that] can make you feel not too good about yourself ... You're opening a can of worms. It's difficult to live with an open can.* (Dean)

Thus, participants here were in accord with theorists about the need to augment mindfulness with particular attitudinal qualities. We might arrange these qualities on a scale, ranging from relatively neutral (e.g., acceptance) to strongly devotional (e.g., reverence), taking in various positive stances along the way (e.g., compassion). Starting with acceptance, men suggested they were exhorted to work towards this by their meditation teachers and in Buddhist books. The idea of acceptance is central to Buddhist philosophy. In particular, while the 'Four Noble Truths' argue that existence is inevitably characterised by suffering, this suffering is thought to be lessened if it is accepted (conversely, resisting it only serves to strengthen it). This view of suffering and acceptance has influenced contemporary forms of therapy, like acceptance and commitment therapy, which explicitly acknowledges its Buddhist origins (Hayes, 2002). Men here saw considerable merit in this philosophy of acceptance. William found that *'one of the reasons why Buddhism makes sense'* is because it encourages one to look at existential *'inevitabilities'*, such as aging or death, *'square in the face, [without] kidding yourself that you might be able to avoid them'*. He felt this was healthier than being in denial.

> *Contemporary society tells us that we should all aspire to being young and beautiful forever. And you can't be. You can't nail down all of those things forever ... and that's what Buddhism keeps reminding us ... To wish for it to be otherwise is to set yourself up for disappointment.*

Participants did not mention a particular practice designed explicitly to cultivate acceptance – unlike compassion (see below) – but just tried to always meditate with this attitude. This was challenging for many, especially given their previous tendencies to disconnect from troubling qualia. For example, Henry talked about being *'an escape artist'*, saying he spent his first five years of meditation *'daydreaming completely'*. Thus, a stance of acceptance certainly did not come easily, but had to be continually worked on. Men had to resist their habitual urge to turn away from difficult qualia, and sought to consciously attend to it with an accepting attitude. This applied to various types of phenomena. For example, Vincent suffered *'incredible pain'* with a foot injury. By *'literally sending the mind'* to the foot and trying to accept the pain, he felt it dissipating (*'It must relax all that area'*). Indeed, this type of mindful acceptance was thought to be behind the success of Kabat-Zinn's (1982) pioneering mindfulness intervention for chronic pain. Others discussed trying to accept their emotional issues. Robert underwent years of therapy trying to get to the 'root' of his recurrent depression. Simply trying to accept these issues, rather than seeking to understand them, was eventually more helpful.

> *I've trawled through that crap too many times. I don't want to be flushed down the toilet again and then go through the swamps, sewers...Acceptance is a big, big thing. Acceptance doesn't mean to say, 'I accept that that's okay', it means you can absorb it into your being, you've transformed the [issue] in some way, so therefore, it's gone.*

Participants also sought to suffuse their attention with more positively qualified attitudes. In particular, many tried to develop a quality known as *metta*, a Pali term translated as 'loving kindness', but which also incorporates compassion and warmth. Men agreed with Kabat-Zinn (2003) that mindfulness should ideally be practised with a feeling of *metta*. Silas: *'It's important to have the right spirit...You can't do mindfulness effectively without emotional positivity, because things will come into mind, and you'll need a perspective on them that's balanced, warm, engaged.'* Helpfully, the FWBO promoted a practice designed to cultivate *metta*, called the *metta bhavana* (bhavana meaning 'cultivation' in Pali). Interestingly, while much of the scientific literature focuses on mindfulness, the *metta bhavana* was given equal weight by the FWBO, these being the two core practices offered in its centres. (It has begun now to be studied, under the name 'loving-kindness meditation', by scholars like Fredrickson and colleagues (2008).) In a five-stage process of guided emotional imagery, practitioners are encouraged to generate positive feelings for themselves – often accompanied by self-affirmative statements (e.g., 'May I be well') – then extend these outwards, first to a close friend, then to increasingly wide circles of people. As Vincent explained:

> *You start with yourself, and then immediate family or friends or loved ones, and then everybody in London, and then everybody in the UK, and then everybody [in the world]. By then it's just a feeling of dispersing this energy anywhere, it doesn't matter who it's to.*

Most men valued the *metta bhavana* highly. It was said to help ameliorate some of the painful contents that emerged in mindfulness, and tempered men's tendencies towards self-criticism (Dean: *'It's about being kind to yourself so you don't beat yourself up'*). Steven called it *'the antidote to the ill-will'*, Dalton described it dramatically as a *'revelation'*, Jimmy suggested it was *'revolutionary'*, and Colin felt it had *'changed the course of my life'*. In particular, men felt it had enabled them to cultivate positive emotions in ways they had previously been unable to. Men appreciated the chance to break free of the restrictive expectations around masculinity – notably the prescription that men should be emotionally tough – that had previously served to discourage them from exploring these kinds of feelings. As Walter put it, *'You definitely feel your heart opening up.'* These findings help illuminate the debate about men's capacity for emotional engagement and expression. Addis's (2008) gendered responding framework made the claim that men are often socialised into a 'restrictive emotionality' affective style. This was supported by men's narratives here of adolescence and early adulthood. However, what we see in relation to the *metta bhavana* is not only the gradual *un*learning of this style, but the extent to which men *appreciated* the chance to develop a more caring emotional style. Dalton described his gradual process of liberation from confining ideas around masculinity that had previously stunted his emotional engagement.

> *The metta bhavana has been really important to me, because it's been helping me to connect with a sense of love and affection, really allowing that more into my life. It's very healing. [Before, caring] didn't fit into my idea of being a man . . . man is more of a warrior, an adventurer . . . For a man to be loving can seem to go against some of the ideas of conditioning . . . It's a work in progress, but it does feel over time I've got more and more in touch with kindness.*

However, the practice could be very challenging. Some men found it highly potent, as trying to generate positivity towards others could bring forth unexpected and powerful emotions.

For example, Jimmy encountered *'strong feelings'* of buried *'grief'* for friends who had died, and he had to turn to therapy to help him process these. Dalton was troubled to uncover anger towards a close friend: *'I couldn't find any positivity. I realised how angry I was with him. It was shocking.'* Given this potency, some men tended to stay away from the *metta bhavana* – Adam experienced *'very strong emotions in the practice'* and didn't necessarily have *'the awareness and the robustness to deal with those fully'*.

Strikingly, some felt that the hardest part of the practice was generating *metta for themselves*. While some scholars suggest that women tend to be more self-critical than men (Neff, 2003), others argue that men collectively have lost self-esteem as social changes have undermined traditional male roles (Ashwin & Lytkina, 2004). Whatever the relative levels of self-esteem of the sexes, results here suggest men may need assistance in cultivating self-compassion, which is a key factor in mental health (Neff et al., 2007). Many men here had long-standing issues around low self-esteem and a propensity towards self-critical thinking. Showing kindness towards themselves was hard, partly because it was unfamiliar – with the practice, Jimmy felt as if he had been *'given permission'* to do something he had *'never done'* before.

> *[It felt] poignant . . . quite an eye opener . . . Just realising that there was such a thing as self-regard, that you could actually practise being . . . kinder to yourself.*

Finally, contemplative attention in meditation can take on even stronger positive dimensions, becoming closer to religious reverence, which Woodruff (2001, p. 63) defines as 'a sense that there is something larger than a human being, accompanied by capacities for awe, respect, and shame'. Although we often associate reverence with theistic religions, this definition implies that it can be directed at anything people feel is 'larger than' the self. For example, we can speak of reverence for nature (Harrison, 2004). Indeed, with the contemporary waning appeal of traditional religions, new forms of worship based around nature have flourished, so-called New Age and Earth spiritualities (Ivakhiv, 2003). Thus, as Goodenough and Woodruff (2001) have identified, meditation can be practised with a spirit of reverence. Moreover, as noted in relation to the Sadhana practice, some Buddhist traditions do revere the Buddha and other figures as deities.

Indeed, discussing deity practices, Jack used religious language to emphasise the importance of *'self-surrender'*, *'reverence'* and *'devotion'* towards these figures. As such, he explained that Buddhism trod a *'middle way'* between theism (*'eternalism'*) and atheism (*'nihilism'*). While rejecting traditional theistic concepts, he explained that Buddhist metaphysics nevertheless proposed that there was a 'force' in the universe – relating to the evolution of consciousness – that could be venerated. In Buddhist philosophy, this force is referred to (in Sanskrit) as the *'Dharma Niyama'*, with Dharma carrying the connotation of 'natural laws', and Niyama meaning 'orders or processes' or 'patternings of reality' (Kang, 2009). Jack had been trying to develop reverence for the Dharma Niyama in his meditations.

> *I started to try and experience more of a devotional element in the meditation, to get me back into a reverential relationship with something else,*

as opposed to just subtly building up my ego ... The Dharma Niyama [is] what you reverence. You could call it God, but [we call it] that level of conditionality that enables you to grow into a Buddha.

Woodruff (2001, p. 63) further suggests that reverence is 'often expressed in, and reinforced by, ceremony'. Indeed, men here discussed ritual ceremonies practised within the FWBO, known as a *'puja'*, a Sanskrit term meaning 'devotional worship' (O'Sullivan, 2001). These ceremonies took a variety of forms, but were generally focused on a central shrine, decorated with images and/or statues of Buddhist figures, together with flowers and incense. The pujas usually involved distinct stages, including devotional chanting from traditional scripture, and opportunities for practitioners to make offerings (e.g., lighting incense) or prayers in front of the shrine. Pujas were a contentious topic: given their strong religious overtones, in light of men's prior rejection of religion, some participants were wary of such activities. Moreover, many had been attracted to Buddhism precisely because they viewed it as dispensing with the trappings of traditional religion. As Ernest said: *'I'm not comfortable worshipping something. It's the antithesis of what I think Buddhism is.'* As such, participants were rather taken aback to encounter such rituals in meditation settings. Some felt uncomfortable, and even refused to join in. William recalled his shock at coming across a puja during his first meditation retreat.

I'd not had any exposure to the Buddhist rituals, I'd just been to meditation classes. Suddenly there was a full on shrine ... with chanting and with people going up doing offerings and bowing, lighting incense. I just thought, 'This isn't what I came here for. I came here for meditation'.... I hated all of that ...I thought, 'I've had enough ritual growing up as a Catholic.'

However, many participants came to appreciate rituals, and the attitude of devotion that they engendered, including some men who had initially been sceptical. As noted above, while men had rejected religion in their youth, some had remained open to finding a sense of spirituality, which pujas duly provided. In articulating why they came to value rituals, many said these offered a sense of meaning. Seligman and colleagues (2006, p. 777) suggest that meaning is found through 'using one's signature strengths and talents to belong to and serve something that one believes is bigger than the self'. Sam articulated this sense of meaning as he recalled a ritual with 80 other men, all in blankets because of the cold, coming together in common purpose:

> *The image which really struck me was all these individual guys with their unique qualities, but all wearing this same red blanket and saluting the shrine. There was something very symbolic about that, a fusion of diversity and unity.*

In describing why the shrine itself was such a meaningful focal point for reflection, Adam saw it as a fecund *'symbol'* of the path he was following (*'It's values, it's a vision, it's a tradition I'm part of, it's the spirit of the Buddha, it's beauty, it's truth'*). Contemplating and bowing to this shrine was a *'mark of respect, recognition and devotion'*. Others found it hard to articulate just why shrines, and rituals conducted around them, affected them so strongly; however, this ineffability was itself part of the appeal. Thus, in these excerpts we can begin to discern part of the broad appeal of meditation/Buddhism. That is, we have discussed above how meditation provided men with resources to engage with their inner world and find ways to constructively manage feelings of distress. However, this section also shows us the ways in which meditation can evoke more elusive and transcendent moments of wellbeing.

> *There's a bit of magic going on that's not entirely explicable. They move me deeply, often to tears...I can't analyse why, and it's something that fascinates me...I love the fact that it's something completely in another realm.* (Grant)

The form of meditation

Finally, the last parameter is the physical form people adopt to meditate, since meditation can be conducted in various postures. Most notably, readers may be familiar with the archetypal 'full-lotus' sitting posture from Buddhist iconography, where the legs are crossed with feet resting on opposing thighs. One of the reasons classically given for this posture is that, anatomically, the triangular formation of the buttocks and knees provides a solid 'base' while allowing deep breathing to be generated by the diaphragm (Ong, 2007). However, the only times men spoke of this posture was to highlight *difficulties* in adopting it, particularly with back problems that impeded their physical flexibility. Thus, while mindfulness can be an intervention for chronic pain (Teixeira, 2008), it was notable that meditation could also generate pain here. Moreover, some men suffered from trying to adopt the 'correct' posture; in 'pushing' their body, they reflected the type of 'macho Buddhism' noted by Scherer (2011). Traditional masculinity idealises the male body as robust, affirmed through physical strength, with weakness a threat to men's gendered identity (Bernardes & Lima, 2010). Here, while men challenged gender norms in many ways, other conventional views persisted, including the need to see oneself, and be seen by others, as physically able. Dustin recalled his battles with this expectation:

> *I sat right in front of the teacher on the cushion and suffered until ... the teacher says, 'Why don't you go and sit on a chair?' Because I wanted to be perfect, [because then] I get approval ... [But] God, the pain in my back was absolute agony ... There's a bit of masochism in there, 'I'm going to be a good body, and hurt myself in the process.' My back was screaming, 'Stop, get me out of this.'*

Over time (and with age), men became less idealistic and rigid about performing the 'correct' posture, allowing themselves to sit in a chair. Additionally, some practices explicitly involved postures other than sitting in a lotus position, such as the body scan, which is conducted lying flat on one's back (Ditto et al., 2006). Indeed, whatever the anatomic merit of the full lotus, it becomes apparent that meditation can be practised in any physical form, and does not even require stillness. Men spoke of walking meditations, trying to be mindful of their ambulatory movements. This practice may be suited to those who have difficulty sitting still, like people with ADHD (Zylowska et al., 2008).

The idea of basing meditation around movement has formed the basis for a diverse range of practices, not least yoga, which as noted is the progenitor of meditation itself. Yoga features physical postures (*asanas*) held for varying durations, accompanied by breathing techniques, that 'unify body and mind' by training one's attention on the body (Sawni & Breuner, 2012). Similarly, Tai Chi involves 'flowing, slow, dance-like movements', where practitioners focus attention on the sensations of respiration and movement (Sandlund & Norlander, 2000). From this perspective, any physical movement can serve as the object of mindfulness. In this way, men showed considerable flexibility in devising their own activities which could generate a meditative state. For example, Ernest struggled to find time to sit formally in his busy routine, but found that breakdancing, his great passion, could generate flow (Csikszentmihalyi, 1990), and so could be meditative.

> *I realised there was meditation to be found there,...because once I'd actually get warmed up and in the music, and it's not a show or a competition...like if I took a little stereo in a field under the sun and start dancing, I would get to a point where I would lose myself in the dance...It would become a hypnotic thing, and my breathing and sense of elation there was unbelievable.*

Going further, any activity, not just movement, can serve as an opportunity for mindfulness. For example, Kristeller and Hallett (1999) developed the idea of eating mindfully as the basis for an intervention for eating disorders. Indeed, men argued that meditation was not a form of escapism, circumscribed from the rest of life. They felt that the point was to try and maintain a mindful stance throughout one's daily activities: '*Awareness should be a thread throughout the day*' (Andrew); '*Live your life being aware, that's the practice*' (Walter). In this spirit, men felt every moment was an opportunity to bring awareness to. Trying to be mindful *in situ* might be called 'meditation-in-action' – a phrase used by Bruce and Davies (2005) in a study of hospice workers who brought mindfulness to bear on their interactions with patients.

For example, Vincent's vision of mindfulness involved '*being aware of everything around me, mindful about my relationship to people...mindful about every aspect of life, and how I live my life*'. This idea of mindfulness-in-action will be important in the next chapter, which looks at the impact meditation had on wellbeing. Meditation not only had the potential to be a rewarding activity in itself, it had a broader impact on how men lived. This is not to suggest that men found it *easy* to be mindful in life. Silas described '*spectacular failures*' in this regard: '*You get off the cushions, and go out in your daily life, you react to the person at the bus stop who's pushed in front of you, and you think, "I wasn't feeling like that about the world and everybody in it half an hour ago!*"' Nevertheless, it was an ideal to aspire to.

> *Driving is good practice. Can you be compassionate with other road users? On the tube in the rush hour, on the telephone...Meditation is all the time. Can you wash up meditatively? How switched on are you? Are you asleep? Be alive, awake.* (Dustin)

Summary

We have seen that meditation is an elastic concept, embracing diverse practices and forms. At the same time though, the essential idea is actually quite simple – meditation is about learning to skilfully deploy one's attention. Within this idea, practices can be differentiated according to four different parameters: *type* of attention deployed (e.g., focused attention, or more mindful 'open monitoring'); *objects* of this attention (e.g., from feelings and thoughts to ideas and images influenced by Buddhism); the *attitude* in which attention is deployed (from acceptance to 'loving kindness' to devotion); and the physical *form* in which one practises (whether sitting still, in movement, or in any daily activity). Having introduced meditation, in the next chapter we look at how these attention skills helped men to find a sense of wellbeing in their lives.

5
Meditation and Wellbeing

The whole of my life I'd just been buffeted around by experience and... had no control over what I was feeling, or what my conscious mind was doing... I realised that if I was able to just work on my mind to the point where it was doing something that I wanted it to do then, then my stress levels just went down enormously. (William)

In the last chapter, we saw how meditation was primarily a system for training attention and awareness, this being the common denominator across the diverse practices featured in the narratives. This chapter picks up the baton by arguing that this development of attention and awareness helped to engender wellbeing in various ways. In Chapter 1, we saw that wellbeing could be conceptualised in multidimensional terms as comprising psychological, social and biological dimensions. Now we shall explore the impact meditation had on these three dimensions. From a psychological perspective, men could better deal with distress. Meditation also helped promote the positive dimensions of wellbeing, i.e., SWB, PWB and EWB. From a social perspective men became more skilled at building relationships. Moreover, by connecting with social groups around meditation, men developed their social capital. Finally from a biological perspective, men were better at engaging in health-promoting behaviours, like cutting down alcohol use. This was partly because of a sense of self-control engendered by their meditation practice, and partly because men were influenced by Buddhist discourses which encouraged such behaviours.

Thus, by developing their attention/awareness through meditation, men became proficient at managing their wellbeing. This is in marked contrast to their narratives of life before starting meditation, as shown in Chapter 3, where many had considerable trouble engaging with their emotional world and managing their feelings. This is also in stark contrast to the way men are commonly viewed in the literature, i.e., emotionally deficient – as reflected in the concept of 'normative male alexithymia' (Levant et al., 2009) – lacking the awareness and skills to engage constructively with their emotions. A helpful way of looking at the impact meditation had on men's wellbeing is through the notion of emotional intelligence (EI). Readers may be familiar with this concept from Goleman's (1995) popularising account. However, the idea originated with Salovey and Mayer (1989), who developed the concept over a series of papers (e.g., Mayer & Salovey, 1997). In contrast to scholars who see EI as a dispositional personality 'trait' (Petrides & Furnham, 2003), their model presents it as an ability amenable to training (Mayer et al., 2008). The narratives support this idea, as men did appear to develop EI through their engagement with meditation.

Mayer and Salovey (1997) conceptualise EI as comprising four hierarchical branches. The 'lowest' branch is emotional awareness and expression. The second branch is the 'emotional facilitation of thought': the 'ability to generate emotions in order to use them in other mental processes' (Day & Carroll, 2004, p. 1444). The third branch concerns an ability to 'understand emotional patterns'. The 'highest' branch is the strategic management of emotions. The lower two branches are labelled collectively as 'experiential EI', which pertains to the information processing of emotional stimuli. The higher two branches are together referred to as 'strategic EI', concerning the strategic management of information processed by the lower branches. The reason the model is conceptualised as hierarchical is that the lower two branches are seen as precursors for the higher two branches. For example, one must first become aware of one's emotions (the first branch) before being able to understand and manage these emotions (the higher branches).

The narratives here support this hierarchical conception of EI. Men did describe developing the respective branches in something approaching a sequential fashion. That said, it was not the case that men gained proficiency at a branch and then 'moved on'. Rather, men *began* working on the branches in their hierarchical order – starting with awareness, i.e., the lowest branch – then continued to work on the earlier branches while also 'stepping up' to the higher branches. As such, this chapter shows how meditation helped cultivate each of the four branches. Thus, this chapter is in four parts, taking each of the EI branches in turn. Each part looks at how the development of that particular branch through meditation helped to facilitate wellbeing, with the three dimensions of wellbeing – psychological, social and physical – running as strands throughout.

Emotional awareness

This first branch requires the least explanation here, since the previous chapter was entirely devoted to the notion that meditation helped develop men's awareness of emotions (and also thoughts, sensations, etc.). This awareness was indeed the first step on their road to emotional intelligence: this was the first ability that men began to acquire through meditation. However, this does not mean men simply attained emotional awareness and then 'moved on' to the other branches. It was a skill that emerged tentatively, in small degrees, and continued to develop over time. As Walter said, reflecting on the way he still had a tendency to '*drift away*' in meditation after ten years practising: '*[E]veryone needs to train. Meditation is just about building awareness.*' As this section explores, enhanced awareness was connected to wellbeing in various ways. First, it enabled men to better tolerate distress. Second, and more positively, awareness sometimes led to sought-after states of mind, like feelings of calm and peace. Third, awareness impacted upon the social dimensions of wellbeing, in particular, enhancing men's interpersonal relationships. These three aspects will be explored in turn.

Firstly, then, enhanced awareness could be helpful when men were under distress, or suffering with unpleasant emotions (e.g., anger). As outlined in Chapter 2, before taking up meditation many participants suffered emotional distress, and even debilitating 'turmoil'. What made the distress so destabilising was that they often experienced themselves as immersed in it – as if caught up in a whirlwind which they could not see clearly. At times, men were even unaware of the extent to which they were in distress. This last point sounds paradoxical, but we can recall the narratives of participants denying their own suffering until they lashed out, perhaps in a violent outburst, sometimes taking themselves by surprise. Indeed, the idea of distress being hidden from men themselves is the very premise of the masked depression framework (Addis, 2008). Thus, participants had been in turmoil, but lacked the capacity to *reflect* upon their distress. However, by paying attention to their inner world in meditation, men were progressively able to enter into a different relationship with their interiority, one of increased '*objectivity*'. This involved observing their thoughts/feelings in a relatively detached, neutral way, referred to in the literature as 'decentring' (Fresco et al., 2007). Silas explained this as:

Being fully engaged with [one's mental content], but not over-identified with it, experiencing it fully, but not being it ... We can see it objectively.

In articulating the value of decentring in the face of negative thoughts/feelings, many men alighted on the notion of greater internal *'space'*. It was as if decentring had an effect of making their phenomenological world, their interiority, literally feel bigger. Dalton described having *'more headspace'*, while Dean spoke of *'distance between you and yourself'*. In experiencing themselves as a bigger, *'stronger vessel'* (Colin), participants were better equipped to cope with negativity by feeling more able to give it space and contain it. This contrasts with men's previous inability to find a way out of their 'turmoil', which led some to contemplate suicide as an escape. Silas: *'In seeing the best and worst of ourselves, we are also bigger to hold it ... The calmness is also like a bigness. One can hold the highs and lows of oneself.'* Thus, while meditation did not necessarily stop negative thoughts/feelings from emerging, by decentring, men were *'less at the mercy of'* these. The increased spaciousness meant that negativity could be kept at more of a distance, and thus felt less close, pressing and immediate.

I [used to] get into some pretty negative internal spaces. It can be very hard. You dive into it. Stepping back from it ... I can see my own states a bit clearer now, I'm not so likely to get buried in them. (Colin)

There is a caveat here: meditation is considered inappropriate for those *currently* suffering with depression. Following Kabat-Zinn's (1982) pioneering MBSR programme, a wealth of similar interventions have emerged, adapted for various physical and mental health problems. The most prominent is Mindfulness-Based Cognitive Therapy (MBCT), designed to prevent *relapse* to depression (Teasdale et al., 2000). The theoretical basis here is the 'differential activation hypothesis': previously depressed people are liable to relapse due to 'dysphoria-activated depressogenic thinking' (p. 615). That is, negative thought patterns associated with previous depressive episodes can be reactivated by negative emotions. By training people's attention, MBCT helps enhance awareness, enabling people to decentre from their cognitions. In turn, this prevents a 'downward spiral' of negative thoughts and worsening negative affect, leading to relapse. In a randomised controlled trial, MBCT plus treatment as usual (patients seeking help from GPs as they normally would) reduced relapse rates for those with three or more previous episodes of depression compared to treatment as usual, with relapse rates of

36 per cent versus 78 per cent (Ma & Teasdale, 2004). As a result, MBCT was approved by the National Institute for Health and Clinical Excellence [NICE] (2004) as a treatment for recurrent depression. Crucially though, the intervention was *unhelpful* for those currently depressed, and was thus contraindicated for such people.

The narratives vividly supported this view of meditation as unhelpful for current depression. Moreover, men's accounts in this area reflect Teasdale and colleagues' (2000) explanation as to why meditation is ill-advised in these circumstances: lacking 'strength' to decentre from negative thoughts as they would usually do, men were drawn into a spiral of 'depressogenic' thinking. Two men in particular discussed recent severe depressive episodes. Walter narrated his as an *'absence of light. Very acute, very intense, very painful ... scared [by] how deep or how dark this absence of light can be ... this deep state of apathy and bleakness.'* Meditation was unhelpful in these circumstances. Depression divested men of the strength to decentre from troubling content as they usually would. Meditation was thus not only unhelpful, but actually counterproductive – it simply made them aware of their negativity, without being able to deal with it. William: *'I'd feel pain, and think, "What the hell's happened to me? I'm a complete wreck." You can get stuck in that. [I lacked] the energy to turn my mind around. I would just experience suffering, and wasn't able to do anything with it.'* Walter emphasised the importance of turning instead to less introspective coping strategies for depression.

> *Don't meditate! I can't emphasise that enough. If you don't have enough light, you get sucked away in the cycle of negative thoughts. It's very unhelpful. Go to the sea, watch TV, that promotes wellbeing.*

However, apart from cases of actual depression, men's developing awareness meant that they were better able to tolerate negative thoughts/emotions. Before starting meditation, men had tended to try and disengage from negative qualia, such as blunting these through alcohol. As noted, such disengagement is a common coping 'strategy' among men (Addis, 2008). When this strategy is explained with reference to masculinity norms around toughness, we make assertions attributing poor mental health outcomes for men to their gender. However, findings here offer a strong counterargument to the prevailing view of men as emotionally deficient: not only are some men emotionally aware, but men who *previously* had been emotionally disconnected can learn to become more aware, in this case through meditation. As we will see throughout this chapter, this awareness helped promote wellbeing in various ways. Regarding negative emotions, subsequent sections show that men learned to actively manage these in various ways. However, even just being aware of these feelings could be helpful. (That said, as noted in the last chapter, sometimes such awareness could also be painful, and had to be augmented by more 'positive' qualities, like compassion.) Sitting in meditation, if negative qualia arose, men found that by just sitting with these, trying to observe them dispassionately, sometimes these became less threatening, or even dissipated altogether.

> *The natural propensity is to go away from suffering and from pain, [but meditation] teaches you how to turn towards it, but not 'I'm going to have to fight with you', but more 'It's OK you're there, I'm not trying to change you, I'm just going to be there.' It just changes the dynamic of it really.* (Henry)

Such awareness was not simply a means for achieving psychological wellbeing in 'negative' terms, ameliorating or muting unwanted states of mind. As noted in Chapter 1, psychological wellbeing can also be conceptualised in 'positive' terms as the *presence* of desirable states or qualities (Hatch et al., 2010). In this respect, men said that increased awareness, and indeed subsequent EI branches, could generate much-sought-after states of mind. The most common feeling described was one of calmness and peace which, when attained, was greatly valued. Men often used the word '*stillness*', which they contrasted with the mental/physical agitation they were more used to experiencing in life. Various analogies were used here. Dean likened the mind to water with '*the surface all churned up*'. In meditation, he could sometimes get '*underneath all the churning*', where '*the deeper you get, the stiller it gets*'. Alternatively, Walter compared the stillness to a garden in the midst of a busy city. Being able to access this calm inner place was helpful during difficult times, allowing him to escape his troubles.

> *I have a place inside my mind that I retreat into, and it's a very safe space. When I was going through this very acute pain, there was relief to have this space.*

When men spoke about stillness, they depicted this as mental, rather than physical, calmness. (Meditation was not generally portrayed as physically relaxing – men more often highlighted experiences of pain, as discussed in the last chapter. This contrasts with the way meditation is often discussed in medical literature as a way to *alleviate* pain; Teixeira, 2008.) Rather, men depicted the stillness as a mental peace. Men frequently experienced the mind as busy. If meditation went well, sometimes the mind *'slowed down'*, became *'exhausted with thoughts'* (Alvin), even reaching a point *'where there is no thought for a while'* (Walter). In articulating their experiences of stillness, men often used the word *'happiness'*. However, they qualified this in revealing ways, using adjectives like *'more refined'* (Adam), *'quieter, softer'* (Ross), *'more satisfied'* (Dalton), *'more pure'* (Dean), or *'strange'* (Walter). Participants also used *'fulfilment'* (Dalton), *'contentment'* (Ross), *'repleteness'* and *'wholeness'* (Silas) to sum up this state. These results align with other studies which suggest that meditation can lead to 'peace and relaxation' (Matchim et al., 2008).

However, the findings here were unusual in two respects. First, such states were relatively rare. While meditation is often portrayed as a state of stillness in academic (Zahourek, 1998) and popular literature (Dillard-Wright & Jerath, 2011), this was a state achieved neither often nor easily in the narratives. It generally took some time to attain, if at all. As Walter said: *'A lot of everyday stuff gets sorted out in the first half hour, and then I can move in ... Some days I get deeper into it, some days I don't.'* Second, the results were unusual in the *strength* of reported SWB, recalling states of contentment which, while relatively rare, were real highlights of their life. Men's experiences thus somewhat challenged the distinction in the literature between SWB (pleasure and satisfaction) and PWB (meaning and growth) (Ryan & Deci, 2001). These narratives suggest that it may not always make sense to present these types of wellbeing as separate, as the most pleasurable/satisfying experiences in men's lives were sometimes the most meaningful.

> *There are moments where I feel just deep, profound satisfaction. Everything is all right as it is, and there's nothing to grasp for, I'm perfectly content just sitting there, being mindful of my experience ... That form of happiness is quite rare, and probably doesn't happen out there in reality, in life.*
> (William)

These new-found skills of awareness were not only deployed within the sedate confines of a meditation sitting. As noted in the last chapter, the point of developing skills in meditation was to deploy these outside such sittings, in life at large. This burgeoning awareness helped men manage their reactions to situations that could otherwise have proved challenging, and which in earlier times might have provoked a more calamitous reaction, like 'lashing out' in aggression. For example, men discussed trying to be mindful in interactions generally, e.g., being attentive to communication dynamics. After Bruce and Davies (2005), we might call this 'meditation-in-action'. This was especially useful in difficult situations. Kris recalled a meeting with his girlfriend he knew in advance would be difficult. Beforehand, rather than pre-rehearsing his arguments, he tried to be mindful so as to enter the encounter in a receptive mode. Rather than responding defensively to the *'hurtful'* content of her speech, he tried to just observe how he was reacting in emotional and somatic terms to the unfolding events. In this way, he kept the lines of communication open so they could work through their issues.

> *[Normally] your body closes and your eyes go down, [but] I felt that in my body, 'I can feel myself closing down, this isn't going to help, I need to stay open here'....I unwound myself from that and opened up, turned and faced her.*

This last excerpt is a powerful illustration of how enhanced emotional awareness was able to impact upon multiple *dimensions* of wellbeing. That is, awareness not only worked upon the psychological dimensions of wellbeing, e.g., allowing men to better tolerate their distress. As Kris's recollection showed, awareness could also promote *social* dimensions of wellbeing. By bringing skills of mindfulness to bear on their social interactions, men's relationships tended to improve. For example, by being more attuned to their own feelings, men were less likely to lash out in reactive ways. Like many, Vincent had previously experienced issues with anger, tending to respond to difficulties with aggressive outbursts. Such externalising responses to distress are common among men, according to the masculine depression framework (Addis, 2008). Crucially, mediation-in-action helped temper this anger. *'Within weeks'* of meditating, Vincent felt *'far more chilled'*. Thus the narratives again show that the issues highlighted by Addis's frameworks are not inevitable, and that men can learn to engage more constructively with emotions, to the benefit not only of themselves, but of those around them. For example, there are links between restrictive emotionality, anger and domestic violence (Schwartz & Waldo, 2003). Thus, that mindfulness may act as a brake on the expression of aggression is noteworthy. As Vincent explained:

> *[There was] a real ability to be aware when anger was kicking in. It's like you've got a third eye watching yourself, saying, 'Don't do that, that's not nice.'*

In this way, greater awareness helped foster more positive interactions. Enhanced awareness meant men were also more attuned to *other* people's thoughts and feelings. Before starting meditation, many men had been relatively disconnected from others – the 'hyperagentic' stance discussed in Chapter 2. In developing mindfulness, men also became more sensitive to emotions in *others*, as predicted by EI theory (Mayer & Salovey, 1997). Increased sensitivity could sometimes be challenging. Prior to meditation, tendencies towards disconnection – internally from troubling emotions, and externally from a difficult environment – were often strategies for dealing with vulnerability. Thus, relinquishing their disconnected stance could render men exposed to vulnerability again. Learning meditation, some men were challenged by a new-found emotional reactivity and lability. Having spent years *'disconnecting'*, Ernest said meditation *'opened the floodgates'*.

> *It was making me sensitive ... I'd be watching an Andrex commercial and I'd burst into tears ... I had to re-adjust. I didn't quite know where I was any more.*

However, men gradually adjusted to their new-found sensitivity, and moreover, grew to greatly appreciate it. Such sensitivity had positive implications for men's relationships, as men found themselves becoming more compassionate. For example, discussing his healthcare work, Kris said: *'I'm more sensitive to people who are in distress, I feel their pain.'* As such, by bringing mindful awareness into their life – within meditation itself, and in their life generally – men were able to generate wellbeing in various ways, from managing distress to promoting more harmonious relationships. Moreover, such enhanced awareness helped men to cultivate the other three EI branches, the next of which is emotional generation of thought.

Emotional generation of thought

Beyond simply being emotionally aware, men were able to promote wellbeing by gradually developing the ability to *generate* positive emotions, which fits the criteria for the second branch of Mayer and Salovey's (1997) model. As Day and Carroll (2004, p. 1444) put it, this refers to the 'ability to generate emotions in order to use them in other mental processes'. In the context of this chapter, the 'other mental processes' in the quote above refers to the cultivation of wellbeing in all its dimensions. First, this means generating emotions in order to alleviate feelings of distress. Second, this means cultivating positive states of mind in their own right, i.e., not simply as part of a strategy for reducing negativity. Thirdly, this means engaging with the social dimensions of wellbeing, such as working towards more harmonious and loving relationships with other people. These three aspects will be considered in turn.

Before considering these three different aspects, it is worth recalling the particular types of meditation practices that are especially associated with the generation of positive emotion. As discussed in Chapter 4, Kabat-Zinn (2003, p. 145) advises practitioners to practise mindfulness with an 'open-hearted, friendly' and 'affectionate, compassionate quality'. However, men often had difficultly imbuing their awareness with the requisite positive spirit. Fortunately, this was remedied in the context of the FWBO where, cognisant of the possibility that practitioners may struggle to practise mindfulness in a spirit of compassion, equal weight was placed on the '*metta bhavana*' practice, with beginners advised to alternate between these. The *metta bhavana*, operationalised in the literature as 'loving-kindness meditation' (Fredrickson et al., 2008), was particularly potent at generating feelings like compassion. (For this very reason, a few men preferred to avoid this practice, finding it hard to handle the strong feelings evoked.) However, many men greatly appreciated its power to produce positive emotions. Some really engaged with the practice on various levels, both cognitive and affective. For example, Silas described bringing skills of creativity into the practice.

> *It's a practice of the imagination. There are wonderful images that I've experienced. For example, sitting and perhaps wondering 'If metta were a colour, what would it be?' And what came was that it would be orange and gold, and slightly sparkling, with a quality of readiness, and so it had a sort of dynamic quality. So the practice was blowing metta-bubbles, which sort of popped over people.*

The practice promoted wellbeing in various ways. First, generating positive feelings had the potential to temper or counteract negative feelings. As Steven said, '*it's the antidote to ill-will*'. This 'antidote' effect corroborates theories of emotion. Theorists suggest that PA and NA are orthogonal constructs – independent processes supervening on different biological mechanisms (Diener & Emmons, 1984). However, in subjective terms, it is proposed that PA and NA are experienced as a single dimension, where each 'dampens' down the strength of the other (Green & Salovey, 1999). Men did indeed find this to be the case. It could be helpful to simply try to replace a negative emotion with a positive one. For example, Walter described the *metta bhavana* as a *'form of self-healing'* that worked to help dissipate feelings of anger. However, it might also be accurate to say the practice worked by bringing positivity to bear on the *source* of their NA, tempering the negativity by cutting it off at the root, so to speak. Walter said that some of his negative thoughts/feelings that arose during meditation concerned feelings of anger, towards himself and towards other people. In the practice, by becoming more compassionate, his anger, irritation or frustration sometimes gave way to understanding and forgiveness. William made a similar point:

> [Through] the metta bhavana I've experienced feelings of interconnectedness and compassion and equanimity, and been able to deal with things that I was really, really angry and hurt about, with people that I was really resentful of.

Thus, learning to generate positive emotions through the *metta bhavana* could be a powerful coping strategy. However, beyond simply managing negativity, the practice opened up more positive avenues of wellbeing, allowing men to experience sought-after states of happiness. For instance, Kris described the great pleasure he got from being creative in his imaginative engagement with the practice (*'Maybe I'm flying with this other person, and I'm like, "Can you feel how good it is to fly?"'*). Aside from indulging his creative side, in a way few other activities appeared to permit, he relished the range of positive qualities he was generating in the practice. He felt this was a wonderful way to use his creativity, especially compared to less fulfilling ends: *'I'm not just creating some idea for a business. I'm being creative in generating goodwill to others and love and kindness ... It's a beautiful thing to be doing with your creativity.'* Tapping into these qualities had an enriching effect. Narratives here align with Fredrickson's (2001) theory of 'broaden-and-build'. This holds that generating positive emotions means people become more open to other sources of wellbeing in their lives – e.g., more open to interacting and cultivating relationships with others. In a similar way, men here found that learning to generate compassion had enriched their lives.

> It's affected my emotional life ... It's made me more supple emotionally, more resilient, in a sort of supple way ... It's changed the course of my life, it's changed the quality of my life. It's more rich than it was. (Colin)

For some men, positive emotions generated or experienced in meditation sometimes gave way to more intensely-qualified positive experiences. (My inclusion of these two terms here – generated and experienced – indicates that this process had an active component, i.e., men explicitly creating emotions, and a passive component, i.e., men being receptive to emotions.) Many men described occasional stronger experiences that went beyond 'ordinary' feelings of compassion or happiness to become something much more charged and powerful. Some used the word '*mystical*' to depict these experiences as mysterious and unusual. Another relevant phrase from the literature is 'anomalous experiences', in the sense of outside the 'standard' range of human experiences. As Peter phrased it, '*qualitatively different from my everyday consciousness*'.

These events were rare occurrences (Dean: '*Once or twice over four years*'). However, they were highlights in men's lives (although they could also be problematic – see below). Here men spoke of intensely positive emotions. Dean recalled an '*absolutely blissful*' experience as '*incredible*'; Robert likened a two-hour '*bliss state*' to '*50,000*' ecstasy tablets; while Jack recalled thinking he wouldn't need sex again ('*It was that good and that positive, I just felt so complete*'). Not all these experiences occurred during formal meditation – some occurred spontaneously, although men attributed them to their practice. Alan described an experience of '*rapture*' while cooking after just two weeks meditating. He explained the episode as '*the natural corollary*' of the '*joyfulness*' he'd been feeling:

> *My hair was standing up on end. Then from inside, a wave of ecstasy, just a complete feeling of love and warmth and more than joy.*

Although these moments are depicted as glimpses, rather than irrevocable shifts to another way of being, men often reported a subsequent change in their view of life. Whilst walking near a monastery, Danny recalled a moment of '*life making sense, a coming together of things in my mind, [with] love being the right way to live in the world*'. Men intimated that such episodes tended to imbue life with a purpose it previously seemed to lack; consequently, many interpreted these as having deep 'spiritual' significance. The concept of 'spirituality' is an elusive one, often characterised as personal and self-defined (Koenig, 2009). Nevertheless, Underwood (1999) suggests that spiritual experiences involve one or more of the following: a feeling of connection with the transcendent (e.g., a higher power); connection with others (e.g., compassion); a sense of meaning (e.g., purpose in life); and a feeling of inner peace. Many such qualities were evident in the narratives. For example, a number of men recalled experiences of 'encountering' a benevolent power which was 'not them' (Peter: *'Something from outside of me'*). One meditation, Sam had a *'vision'* of a sphere *'hovering'* in his chest.

> *It was made of light, golden and vibrating, full of energy...I felt confident that if I'd manage throughout my life to make a path to reach that source, and was able to tap into it, everything would be fine...my spiritual development would unfold naturally.*

Some spiritual experiences were religious in nature. Here, the cognitive and aesthetic aspects of experiences were influenced by the particular tradition within which men practised. These findings relate to a perennial debate in the literature on spirituality. Constructionist theorists hold that spirituality is not about numinous experiences, but the adoption of particular discourses that mark one out as 'spiritual' (Popp-Baier, 2002). Conversely, positivist theories understand spirituality in terms of actual anomalous experiences (Coyle, 2008). Both perspectives were supported here. Men genuinely had potent anomalous episodes, and yet their experience and interpretation of these was inextricably coloured by the contextual framework in which they practised. For example, Sam recalled an intense experience generated by a visualisation practice given to him by his teacher (*'Visualise a white lotus flower, and then destroy it'*). This practice had the effect on Sam of feeling a sense not only of his absent teacher's presence, but also the presence of his teacher's teacher, and even figures further back in the 'lineage'. He recounted an overwhelmingly positive sensation of *metta* being 'showered' upon him by these venerable figures within his specific Buddhist tradition.

> *[I] suddenly [felt] the presence of my teacher's teacher...I could see him clearly, quite sharply, floating in this blue sky...He was full of metta towards me, very, very strong...As that continued the energy changed into a rain of diamonds or golden streams of nectar...both hard as diamond as well as soft as honey, just streaming down on my head...I just bathed in this light that came down as a blessing.*

Before leaving the topic of mystical experiences, it is crucial to mention an important caveat. Some intense experiences could be so potent and emotionally charged that they were difficult to understand. Sometimes the consequence was nothing more serious than inflated pride. For instance, Danny recalled an episode (*'Literally being thrown around in my body'*) which he thought signified he would *'get enlightened'* imminently. In retrospect, his *'ego got carried away'*: *'I remember telling the guys, "Have I got a story for you" .... I got intoxicated and felt special.'* He felt this was understandable given that he'd *'never had anything like that before and didn't know how to interpret it or what to do with it'*. For some though, such experiences undermined their sense of reality. Adam recounted early episodes that were so *'far outside'* his *'usual experience'* as to be *'disorienting'*. An *'out of body'* sensation was *'alienating and disturbing'*, and left him feeling *'sick'*. Even a blissful experience was *'frightening'*: he felt compelled to scrabble around touching objects afterwards to reassure himself he was real (*'It felt like I'd disappeared into some ethereal sort of realm. I wanted to ground myself'*). Most troubling was when he attempted the advanced Six element practice alone as a beginner. As noted in Chapter 4, without guidance, he was enveloped by a sense of *'meaninglessness'*.

> *I crashed, I ended up lying on the floor sobbing, because I had a really strong sense of impermanence without the context, without the positivity. The crushing experience of despair was very strong... You just feel like you don't exist, you're just nothing, there's nothing really there. It's nihilistic, pretty terrifying.*

In a small number of cases, participants suggested that these potent disorienting experiences in meditation were linked to severe adverse psychological effects, including reality-testing, depersonalisation and despair. Three men linked these adverse experiences to subsequent states of psychosis, with two sectioned for psychotic breakdowns. Meditation is recognised as inappropriate for those at risk of psychosis (Lustyk et al., 2009). However, there is little research on the potential for meditation to precipitate such consequences in the general population (Dobkin et al., 2012). This lacunae fits in with a general trend in the literature: Irving et al. (2009, p. 65) suggest that amidst the enthusiasm to explore the potential benefits of meditation, a 'striking limitation' here is the 'absence of research on potentially harmful or negative effects'. A few case studies have linked meditation to adverse psychological effects – Kuijpersa and colleagues (2007), Yorston (2001) and Shapiro (1992) – including anxiety, depression and psychosis. However, Perez-De-Albeniz and Holmes (2000) contend that such case studies generally do not adduce causality, since these do not disentangle the effects of meditation from pre-existing psychological issues.

Causality cannot be ascertained in this study either. However, although one man admitted to mental health problems before taking up meditation, the remaining five mentioned no prior experience of such problems. Moreover, four of these believed their adverse experiences had been directly caused by meditation. It must be emphasised though that these men felt their problems had been due to meditating incorrectly and/or to lacking peer guidance to help them interpret powerful experiences. They still viewed meditation positively, some even attributing significance to their experiences, constructing them as potent moments of insight. Narratives here thus support the concept of post-traumatic growth (Tedeschi & Calhoun, 2004), where traumatic events can induce positive changes, like gratitude for life. Still, these men's stories reinforce the idea that meditation has the potential to be a powerful technique – a *'power-tool'* in Adam's words – and as such must be respected and used with caution, even in non-clinical populations. Even potent experiences that are generally experienced as positive can be challenging (e.g., destabilising one's worldview). Moreover, the narratives emphasise the need to augment an ability to generate strong emotions with skills in terms of *understanding* these emotions. Indeed, such understanding is the third branch of Mayer and Salovey's (1997) model of EI, and will be considered further in the following section.

Before turning our attention to emotional understanding, it is worth noting the impact of this second branch of EI upon the social dimensions of wellbeing. As suggested by Fredrickson's (2001) broaden-and-build theory, the ability to generate positive emotions improved men's relationships in manifold ways. It was not simply that men felt more compassionate to others during the meditation practice; it had potent and durable effects in actual interactions. Such developments are striking. As outlined in Chapter 2, before taking up meditation, many men had been relatively disconnected from those around. Indeed, in the literature men are viewed as having smaller social networks and fewer close friendships than women (Davidson, 2004). Taking Bakan's (1966) distinction between agency and communion, Wilber (1995) refers to this emphasis on individuality as 'hyperagency'. Some theorists attribute such hyperagency to masculine norms around independence and invulnerability (Pollack, 1998). However, whilst men previously endorsed and enacted this 'lone man' stance, in retrospect, they felt that they had suffered because of it. For example, John described his previous isolation as generating a sense of fear. Through meditation, he came to value feeling a greater sense of connectivity with others.

It's important to do the metta bhavana, because it gives you a sense of being alright ... Fear can arise because one thinks one is alone or separate ... but the metta bhavana is like a vision of what it's like when you're not separate. You feel very connected, it's nourishing the act of living connectiveness that exists.

Moreover, beyond this valued yet abstract notion of feeling more *'connected'*, generating positive emotions towards others had the practical effect of developing men's relationships. This occurred in various ways. For example, empathy and compassion are seen as comprising affective and cognitive dimensions, where people can appreciate, understand and respond to another's emotional state (Baron-Cohen & Wheelwright, 2004). These skills were cultivated by men here, as discussed below in relation to the third branch of the EI model, emotional understanding. However, aside from empathic understanding, simply working on bringing prosocial emotions like kindness to bear on social interactions had a powerful effect on men's relationships. For example, Colin felt his early years of marriage were difficult because he was *'basically trying to get [his wife] to change to be something that she wasn't'*. However, by cultivating kindness, he was able to be more accepting of her, which meant they argued less. Silas discussed the positive effect of acting upon prosocial qualities generated in meditation: *'[If you] experience a sense of wanting to help or be kind to somebody, just do it.'* Steven described preparing for potentially difficult encounters at work. He found it helped to first get himself into a positive state of mind regarding his impending protagonist.

If you knew they were coming [for a meeting], you'd sort it out the morning before, put them in [the metta bhavana], so when they come you're already thinking positively about them ... Then I was listening to them much better and [being] more receptive.

So far, we have seen the way meditation enabled men to develop the first two EI branches – emotional awareness, and ability to generate emotions – known collectively as 'experiential' EI. These 'lower-level' skills were conducive to wellbeing in various ways. Going further though, men also began to develop the two 'higher' branches of EI, known collectively as 'strategic' EI: emotional understanding, and the strategic management of emotions. We will consider these in turn, beginning with understanding.

Emotional understanding

We are now moving into the third of the EI branches, emotional understanding. This refers to 'the ability to understand and reason about emotional information and how emotions combine and progress' (Day & Carroll, 2004, p. 1444). As indicated above, it would be inaccurate to present these branches as a series of discrete steps; rather, as men progressed in meditation, they continued to work on all four branches simultaneously, each branch interacting with and reinforcing the others. That said, there is validity in the idea of men *beginning* to develop each branch in something approximating sequential fashion. For example, one can appreciate that being aware of emotions might be a prerequisite for understanding those same emotions.

Thus, as detailed in the previous chapter, men began their meditation career by learning to simply pay attention to their inner world. As their attention/awareness developed, they began to infuse this attention with positive attitudinal qualities, as outlined in the second section above. Then, with repeated observation of the internal workings of their mind, men began to gain some understanding of their mental dynamics. This included an appreciation of recurrent thought patterns, the on-going creation of self-identity, and the phenomenology of emotions (e.g., the way feelings dynamically shade and shift into one another). As with the first two branches, this understanding helped men cultivate wellbeing in various ways, enabling them to manage negativity, develop 'positive' states of mind, and enhance the social dimensions of wellbeing. These different aspects will be explored in turn.

First, greater understanding helped men cope with negative thoughts/feelings. In this respect, there was particular emphasis on two forms of understanding in the narratives: understanding the phenomenology of negativity and understanding its origins/reasons. With the former, men found it helpful to gain some insight into the dynamics of their negative states. Beyond just becoming aware of negative qualia (the first EI branch), men began to appreciate *patterns* of such qualia. As Silas said: '*I became more aware of how I habitually thought. [We're] just a bag of habits really.*' In this way, men began to notice recurrent patterns of negative thoughts. Appreciating this recurrent nature helped men to decentre from them. Rather than seeing such thoughts as 'true' statements – e.g., about the self – that must be believed, men could view these more as dysfunctional mental 'tics', unfortunate quirks of their mental processing that did not warrant respect or attention. For example, Terry had experienced depression in the past. Echoing cognitive theories of depression, he linked this to a tendency to ruminate on negative self-referential thoughts (Teasdale, 1988). Through understanding his proclivity to rumination, he was less drawn into it.

> *Rather than going off down some spiral into a pit of despair, drawing all sorts of conclusions about myself, [like] 'I'm worthless', now I just stop it there and go, 'I'm doing that again.' Not buying into it. Not giving it any currency.*

Moreover, beyond just understanding the recurrent patterns of negativity, men began to gain insight into the temporal dynamics of such negativity. In particular, they began to appreciate the *transiency* of mental phenomena, their fleeting, ephemeral nature. As Silas said: '*We can see the truth, that mental states are not permanent, they're changing and developing.*' Before taking up meditation, men suggested that in the midst of a negative state, it had the potential to feel intractable. This misapprehension increased the burden of such states, since it felt as if they were permanent and enduring. Through an understanding of transiency, men were given succour by '*just knowing it will pass*' (Terry). Moreover, this understanding reined in men's previous tendencies to want to *react* to their negative qualia. As Vincent vividly expressed it, this meant not '*just headlessly being this emotional animal that's blown by the wind*'. In this way, while men still experienced negative qualia, they were less perturbed by these, reassured by a sense of light at the end of the tunnel.

> *You can sit with hate ... fear, loneliness, longing, sadness. You know it will pass ... Whereas before I didn't have the awareness, I thought it would last forever.* (Dustin)

In many narratives, this understanding of phenomenology became augmented by a second, deeper form of understanding: of the *origins* of negativity. Beyond simply appreciating the dynamics of negative mental states, men developed insight into why these states occurred in the first place. For example, some men observed that there are not just feelings, but feelings about feelings, described by Denzin (1985) as 'meta-feelings'. Although negative feelings may be unavoidable, having a negative meta-feeling *about* the negative feeling – feeling bad about feeling bad – compounded the problem. In relation to this, a few men referred to the Buddhist idea of the 'two arrows': although they couldn't prevent negative feelings from occurring (the first arrow), by accepting them, at least they could avoid adding to them (the second arrow). As William said: *'There's the immediate thing that causes you to suffer, then there's all the suffering created in thinking about it. That second bit of suffering is something I can work on.'* Thus men understood that they were compounding their suffering by creating story-lines around negative events and replaying these continually in their mind. Realising this, men endeavoured to cease adding 'fuel to the fire'.

> *When I ruminate, when I run these conversations, I increase my irritation. It's painful to me ... Some suffering is inevitable ... but we heap loads more on top, just through the way we respond.* (Silas)

Men also made intricate observations around the way suffering was linked to a person's sense of identity. Discussion around the nature of the 'self' is central to literature on meditation and Buddhism (Wilber, 1995). Much attention is paid to the idea of the 'ego', a term popularised by Freud (1949) (although the credit should really go to Freud's English translator, Strachey, who chose the Latin term to express the German word for 'I' that Freud himself used). Without wishing to over-simplify a vast and contested field of enquiry, a key idea is that negative states of mind are the product of clinging to the idea of an ego. In this context, the 'ego' may be thought of as the 'belief' that one exists as a separate self, i.e., a fixed, stable, discrete entity enduring over space and time. This notion of a fixed identity has been challenged from many quarters, not only in Eastern systems of thought, but by Western thinkers too. For example, the philosopher Dennett (1990) views the notion of a fixed self as a cognitive illusion created by a potent combination of memory and language (e.g., grammatical constructions involving first person pronouns). He thus describes the self as the 'centre of narrative gravity'. This idea has a venerable pedigree in Western philosophy (Gallagher, 2000). For example, Hume (1739) saw the self as a product of the temporal succession of fleeting subjective impressions being tied together by the imagination.

Similar conceptions of the self abound within Buddhist literature. However, what is striking in Buddhism is that, whereas Western philosophical frameworks aim simply to elucidate this kind of theory of the self, Buddhism strives to help people *experience* it. That is, meditation can be used as a technology that allows the insubstantiality of self to be directly apprehended. As Epstein (1988, p. 62) put it, in meditation 'the "I" experience is revealed to be a constantly changing impersonal process, increasingly insubstantial the more it is examined.

As a result the self-concept that was once experienced as solid, cohesive and real ... becomes increasingly differentiated, fragmented, elusive and ultimately transparent.' Similar ideas were found in the narratives. It was common to hear men say the ego or the self was an *'illusion'*, and that they were trying to *'surpass'* it or *'break it down'* (Peter). Mirroring the description proffered by Epstein, men described probing their sense of identity in meditation. Through this process, some came to endorse the perspective outlined by Hume (1739), viewing the self as just an ever-changing stream of qualia. For example, Peter explained how he questioned his sense of self during meditation, and found himself 'creating' a sense of self.

> *I just go in cold, [asking], 'What is the self?' ... I can notice myself making a self ... So for example, I notice I experience pride that I've got a full head of hair ... That's me attaching to a sense of self ... I then use that to see how I'm creating an illusory sense of self.* (Peter)

Thus, men talked about developing greater understanding of the nature of the self, including the 'ego'. The significance of this understanding vis-à-vis wellbeing is that, in Buddhism, the ego is held responsible for much of people's suffering. Walter felt the ego fluctuated wildly between the *'flush of triumph'* (self-pride at life going well) and the *'laying of blame'* (self-condemnation at life going badly). Thus, the ego was discussed as if a kind of fragile fortress, always vulnerable to attack, always needing to be bolstered by ego 'boosts'. As Ali put it vividly, *'It's like a ravenous rabbit. It's a monster, it's a beast. It just wants to be fed.'* Men then linked this continual struggle to protect and *'feed'* the ego to unhappiness. For example, Michael felt most dysphorias were due to *'self-pre-occup[ation]'*: *'At one end of the scale you get depression, one of the major symptoms of which is self-absorption ... At the other end of the scale you get something like violence, which is an ego trying to defend itself.'* As such, men argued that by reducing their 'self-pre-occupation', they could alleviate some of the negative thoughts/feelings generated by their sense of self. For example, Ali described previously getting distressed at various failures in life. For him, trying to become 'egoless' meant developing a sense of perspective, which he found to be an effective strategy.

> *I'm trying to be egoless ... It's a sense of proportion? You're just another dot in the universe, you know what I mean? In the scheme of things, it doesn't matter. It's like, if I'm not there, the sun will still rise.*

Thus, coming to understand the self as 'constructed', and trying to view events from a less egocentric perspective, could be effective in alleviating distress. For some men though, this kind of understanding led to more strongly qualified positive states of mind. Here we are back again in the realm of 'mystical' or 'anomalous' experiences, states of mind that were radically different from 'ordinary' everyday states. For example, in the previous chapter we recounted an experience Sam had while immersed in the Six element practice. In this, the sight of ducks drinking blood challenged his concept of a duck ('*[Its] definition exploded in my brain*'). He found this sudden conceptual re-evaluation turned reflexively upon himself: '*I thought, "If it doesn't have a fixed identity, is this the case [for me]?" ...I was a changed person, I've never been able to think about things in the same way.*' In terms of positive effects of such shifts in understanding, Sam's assertion that the experience helped alleviate his anxieties around death bears repeating.

> *For a few days all my fear to die had lifted ... Nothing exists as a thing and then dies and disappears, just constantly a stream of change, one thing moves into another. Being more in touch with that in meditation ... did loosen up some of my anxieties.*

Finally, enhanced understanding helped men cultivate the social dimensions of wellbeing by giving them greater insight into *other people's* emotional dynamics. Here, men built upon the social skills depicted above in relation to the first two branches, such as being mindful in interactions. These skills were augmented by a better *understanding* of others, and of how to interact in ways conducive to wellbeing. As noted above, men developed prosocial qualities like compassion through meditation, especially the *metta bhavana*. However, these qualities do not simply involve expressing positive emotions; they comprise affective and cognitive dimensions, including understanding others' emotional states (Baron-Cohen & Wheelwright, 2004). Men felt that practising compassion in the *metta bhavana* functioned as an effective exercise in learning to take another's *perspective*. There were parallels here with Buber's (1958) distinction between 'I–It' relationships (others viewed just as means to an end) and 'I–Thou' relationships (others valued as ends in themselves). For example, William felt that the practice had '*open[ed] up this world of possibilities about how you can relate to people, how equal we are, how everybody is as much a human-being, worthy of value as I am*'. Other men had similar narratives of becoming less self-occupied and more understanding of others.

It helps me to see other people, complete strangers, as human beings, rather than just people who are in my way, or something, and to have a bit more perspective, be a bit less selfish. (Dean)

This sense of understanding cultivated through perspective-taking enabled men to develop better relationships in various ways. Men enjoyed having greater insight into communication dynamics generally, which meant they interacted more effectively with others. For example, Andrew was more sensitive to the way he gave advice in the workplace, understanding that if he was *'a little bit more gentle with it'*, then his audience would likely be more receptive to it. Others recalled bringing their understanding to bear specifically on difficult social situations. For instance, Steven suggested that if people acted in ways that he perceived as unfriendly or aggressive, he had become able to defuse his negative reaction to such people by dwelling on the possible causes of such behaviour: *'When somebody does do something [bad], I think..., "They're probably doing it because they're not happy, because they're stressed".'* Other men dealt with negative reactions to other people by reflecting on the consequences of *expressing* this negativity in an unskilful way. Grant still got *'pissed off'* at people, but now had greater insight into the futility of his anger.

> *Righteous indignation is absolutely useless. It doesn't get you anywhere. Sure, you're right – he's done something to piss you off. But are you going to be able to alter his behaviour? No. So, you've got to accept that and forgive...I've learned to recognise that irritation and anger and self-righteousness that arises in me much earlier and just say, 'Look, let's stop.' It doesn't do any good just turning it over in your mind and basically egging it on.*

What is particularly interesting about this excerpt is how Grant described using his emotional understanding to choose a particular course of action in this situation, i.e., making a positive decision to forgive. Thus, we can see how the third EI branch shades subtly into the fourth, namely, the strategic management of emotions.

Strategic management of emotions

Finally, we reach the fourth branch of Mayer and Salovey's (1997) EI model, the ability to 'moderate' emotions in oneself and others. This

is the culmination of the previous branches. Having cultivated awareness and understanding, men developed the ability to actively *change*
their emotions. This skill can be located within a wider framework
of self-regulation theory, encompassing regulation of motivation, cognition, social interaction and behaviour (Carver & Scheier, 1998). In
this theory, people are volitional agents, capable of conscious, motivated decision making, planning and goal-directed determination. Thus,
emotional management concerns self-regulation of emotion, using cog-
nitive/behavioural strategies to evoke, suppress or alter emotions. The
idea of emotional management does not only find its expression in the
EI model. The concept of emotion regulation, associated with Gross
(1999), pertains to 'monitoring, evaluating, and modifying emotional
reactions, especially their intensive and temporal features' (Thompson,
1994, pp. 27–28). Similarly, emotion work refers to 'the act of trying to
change in degree or quality an emotion or feeling' (Hochschild, 1979,
p. 561). These overlapping concepts found their expression in the narratives. Men learned to consciously affect their emotional dynamics,
changing how emotions were experienced and responded to.

The key word here is *control*. In the past, men felt somewhat at the
mercy of their internal experience – *'headlessly being this emotional animal that's blown by the wind'*, in Vincent's memorable phrase. Through
meditating, men began to feel more in charge of their emotional
dynamics. As with the other branches, this burgeoning skill promoted
wellbeing in various ways, whether managing negative emotions, promoting positive states of mind, or enhancing relational wellbeing.
Taking first the management of negativity, building on their emotional
awareness and understanding, men developed skills to actively *'work'*
with internal feelings. Here, meditation was constructed as a process of
acquiring helpful *'tools'* (Kris), enabling *'working on ourselves with ourselves'* (Silas). We saw glimmers of such tools in the earlier branches.
For example, 'decentring' did not simply mean being aware of internal
experience, but *'stepping back'* from it, learning to detach oneself. In this
notion of stepping back, we see men beginning to exert active control
over their mental life. In this fourth branch, this kind of control became
more conscious, willed and skilful.

The forms of emotional management and control discussed in this
section were not only deployed within meditation practice. As with
the other branches, while these skills were literally 'practised' within
meditation sittings, the ideal was to harness these skills in general life.
Before reflecting on the various ways in which men described managing their emotions, it is worth appreciating the general phenomenology

of this sense of control, i.e., how did it *feel* to be able to exert influence over one's emotional life. The notion of 'meditation-in-action' was introduced above. In doing this, men enjoyed a new-found ability to critically reflect *in the moment* on their own actions. Soon after taking up meditation, Vincent recalled *'a real ability to be aware when anger was kicking in. It's like you've got a third eye watching yourself.'* With this ability to reflect, men found themselves becoming less reactive: Silas described it as a temporal 'gap' opening up *'between feeling and acting'*; Ernest called it a *'slowing down of myself'*. Thus, while situations could still provoke negative impulses, men felt they had more 'time' to keep these in check. Steven recalled constantly getting angry with people at work (*'My mouth would be shouting before I'd even noticed'*). After he began meditating, a *'thinking pause'* began to appear.

> I'd think, 'Last time I shouted I didn't enjoy it, and it didn't do any good anyway, so I won't shout this time' .... Once I was aware of that, it opened up and opened up ... Now this gap is so big, I can't get angry any more, nothing really touches me.

Connected to this sense of control is a related theme of freedom and choice. Men here had an interesting perspective on free-will: rather than either having or not having it, they tended to see themselves as experiencing *degrees* of freedom. Before meditation, they often reacted automatically to situations. While they still had residual 'tendencies' to respond in particular ways, they enjoyed greater freedom of choice now. William: *'[I felt] incredibly liberated ... You have some choice about how you react, rather than an automatically programmed response.'* Thus, we can trace a pattern of phenomenological development here: mindfulness-in-action generating the ability to reflect critically on one's actions/reactions as they are occurring; this reflectiveness reducing men's reactivity; and lower reactivity enabling greater freedom of choice in how to respond. This enhanced freedom was then coupled with the kind of emotional understanding discussed above to produce more effective responses. As part of the process of acquiring insight into their own emotional dynamics, men began to appreciate how particular cognitive/behavioural strategies could produce desired outcomes. Freedom of response then meant that they were better able to *enact* these strategies as appropriate.

One of the ways in which this control occurred was in the skilful deployment of attention. Beyond simply *'stepping back'*, men cultivated the ability to deal with negative thoughts and feelings by selectively focusing their attention. For example, men discussed learning to move attention towards sensations in the body through a meditation called the 'body scan'. This involved going *'over each part of the body with your mind'* (Robert), trying to be aware of visceral feelings in each area. While in itself the practice was depicted as pleasant, it was also a strategy for dealing with negativity. Shifting focus to bodily sensations, attention became diverted from troubling thoughts. Men described being affected by complex cognitions, like worries or regrets, which had the power to generate distress. One way of trying to deal with such cognitions was by trying to adopt a strategy of *'living in the now'* (Terry). As men explained, focusing attention on the body was an expedient way of doing so.

The notion of a 'present-orientated' time perspective being a route to wellbeing is common currency in popular self-help and spiritual literature (Tolle, 2004). The idea that people tend towards different time perspectives is also addressed in psychological literature, particularly in the work of Zimbardo and colleagues (e.g., Zimbardo & Boyd, 1999). However, in that context, a 'balanced-time' perspective, involving past, present and future considerations, is deemed most conducive to wellbeing (Boniwell et al., 2010). In the narratives though, the emphasis was very much on the desirability of a present-time perspective. (This possibly reflects the influence of discourses from self-help books in meditation circles; indeed, some men specifically mentioned the Tolle book cited above.) Men argued that one of the benefits of trying to adopt a present-focused time orientation was that it divested negative future- or past-oriented thoughts of their salience. Focusing on the body was an effective way to do this. As Dean put it, *'Your body isn't thinking of the future or the past.'* John described relieving himself of negative thoughts in a meditation.

> *I just paid attention to the sensations in my chest...After a while I had let go of my thoughts...that were giving rise to my suffering. Then I just felt happier.*

Conversely, some argued that rather than a means of escaping troubling qualia, focusing on the body was a good way of *engaging* with them, but at a physical level. Here, men described coming to understand emotions as embodied, i.e., having a somatic aspect. As Dustin put it, *'difficulties manifest as physical stuff, become somatised'*. For example, one aspect of anxiety might be visceral sensations of churning in the abdominal area. The idea that emotions have a somatic dimension is well-recognised in the literature (Barrett & Lindquist, 2008). Of special relevance here is that men learned to actively engage with this dimension as a way of dealing with negative cognitions. Rather than facing these directly, men could engage them indirectly by focusing on their somatic manifestations, which could be less threatening. For example, Walter recalled feeling upset after an argument, experienced somatically as his *'chest closing in'*. In meditation, he tried to become mindful of sensations there, and the negative emotion eventually *'dissolved'*:

> *If one is deeply troubled...you can't treat the emotional pain with such immediacy. So you treat the physical pain to alleviate the physical manifestations.*

This was a radical new approach to dealing with negativity. As noted in previous chapters, before taking up meditation, men often sought to blunt or escape from negative feelings. Now, they saw the value of not only trying to *'stay with'* such feelings, but trying to actively probe them with a stance of benevolent curiosity. Here again we see challenges to essentialist ideas that men are inevitably poor at engaging with their emotions. Such news is succour to all who hold out hope of helping men change for the better. However, of particular value here is that rather than simply exhorting men to change, here we have identified a specific practice that can promote the desired result, i.e., meditation. For example, Henry explained a method called *'focusing'*, which *'aims at allowing your body to tell you what's going on'*.

> *You just look at whatever it is you're not feeling very satisfied with, and try to engage with it as a sensation, just kind of giving it a voice really, entering into a dialogue with it. The principle is that [it's] like you were sitting on a bench with an old friend, where you don't really need to console it or anything, just be there...It just changes the dynamic of it really...It can be very releasing.*

Many men discussed the wider value of re-connecting with their bodies, saying this opened up possibilities for cultivating a more positive sense of wellbeing. In Chapter 2, we explored how, before starting meditation, encouraged by masculinity norms, participants had become disconnected from their emotions. Some men recalled that this disconnection extended to bodily experience in general, with a tendency to live *'in the head'*. As Ross put it, *'We escape into a mental bubble of conceptual understanding.'* As with emotional disconnection, this type of 'disembodiment' has been linked to masculinity in the literature. For example,

popular opinion often constructs different types of psychological processes as being gendered in some way. For example, 'rationality' and
cognitive mentation generally are typically seen as more masculine;
and 'intuition' and 'felt knowledge' generally viewed as more feminine
(Ross-Smith & Kornberger, 2004).

Thus, many men lamented that they had become somewhat 'cut off'
from their body – Harry called this *'our tragedy'*. Intriguingly, some
said that mindfulness meditation could actually *reinforce* this bodily
disconnection. Grant described it as sometimes producing *'an alienated experience where it's all in the head'*. Men thus valued becoming
re-acquainted with their embodied self through practices like the body
scan. The narratives here extend the enlarged 'headspace' theme highlighted above – where men were better able to cope with distress as their
mind felt like a bigger/stronger *'vessel'* – incorporating a wider visceral
expanse. Colin felt he had found *'a whole new dimension'* through bodily awareness, and now felt *'a whole lot more spacious'*. Andrew indicated
that such re-embodiment generally felt good: *'I am immediately happier
if I bring myself into my body and . . . create more space for everything.'*

In addition to the skilful deployment of attention, men described
other cognitive 'tools' they had acquired which helped to manage negativity. One technique involved asking questions about the issue at hand.
Such questioning is a core process of certain forms of psychological therapy, like cognitive behavioural therapy (Beck et al., 1979). In this, the
therapist seeks to challenge the negative self-referential thoughts that
might underlie a client's psychological problems through a process of
Socratic questioning (Overholser, 1993). What is striking here is that
men developed such strategies autonomously. For instance, some used
the example of feeling angry after an argument. Adam said this process of questioning included challenging the legitimacy of his thoughts
about the incident (*'Asking "Is this actually true?"'*). John would critique
the narrative he had built up around it (*'[I realise] it's a story I'm telling,
as opposed to reality'*). Others described querying the use of their anger
(Grant: *'It doesn't get you anywhere'*) and who it affected (Silas: *'No-one is
experiencing that pain except for [me]'*).

> *[I] challenge that thought as a reality. Then sometimes it disappears. I'm
> much better able to adjust my mood swings, and not be fooled by my own
> psychology'.* (Robert)

Learning to adopt a detached perspective through meditation, men
could critically reflect upon their own 'psychology'. In this way, men

functioned as their *own* therapist. This has parallels with a study by Ridge and colleagues (2008): through meditation/prayer, patients with HIV created a dialogue with an 'absent counsellor', which alleviated distress. Another therapeutic strategy that men in the current study enacted upon themselves was adopting different *'perspectives'* that altered the significance of their troubles. For example, Ali spoke above about developing a sense of insight into his own relative unimportance in the world. He tried to respond to distress by reflecting on this insight (*'It's a sense of proportion. You're just another dot in the universe … In the scheme of things, it doesn't matter'*). Conversely, Alvin sought to put his troubles in the context of other things for which he could feel grateful (*'I've got lots of blessings I can feel thankful for, [which] gives a bit of perspective'*). As with questioning, men indicated that this 'perspective-taking' was a skill that had been acquired or developed with meditation. Vincent described a new-found ability to cognitively defuse his negative reactions through rational analysis:

> *It's just this ability to rationalise. [Before] I would've let it fester. It would've upset my whole evening. [Now] I'm able to step back that much quicker and be analytical, seeing things for what they are.*

Other coping strategies were behavioural and externally directed, like exercise or talking with others. As Danny said: *'[T]here's things that I do that I know help me to keep sane and positive, like running, trying to make time for friends.'* Of course, before taking up meditation, men had various coping strategies that worked for them to some extent, even if ultimately these were experienced as maladaptive. However, the crucial point here is that, through meditation, men were able to *strategically* manage their emotions by skilfully choosing the appropriate response. That is, men described being aware of a range of strategies at their disposal to help manage stress/distress. Men specifically linked this awareness to their meditation practice. That is, mindfulness was not only a helpful response in itself to difficult situations. Through being mindful, men felt they were better able to select other coping responses as appropriate. Meditation-in-action thus engendered what self-regulation theorists call meta-coping abilities (Carver & Scheier, 1998), i.e., knowing how to skilfully choose from different strategies, and using these to help manage emotions in an effective way.

> *I still get bad moods, but I'm much more able to know what to do. Before I wouldn't do anything about it. I'd just carry on getting upset, being stuck*

in it. But now I know I've got ways to get out of it... There's all sorts of things you could try... It's so easy to think one's the victim of one's own mind, but... we're in the driving seat. (Jack)

Ironically, having developed emotional management through meditation, these skills meant men knew when to *refrain* from meditation. In the last chapter, we saw that meditation could be inappropriate for states of low mood, as lacking the strength to decentre, it could actually increase distress. Other men also said meditation could be an inappropriate strategy for states of anxiety, since it had the potential to increase men's sense of vulnerability to the source of their anxiety. Adam found that *'getting into deep meditation just made you more sensitive, when actually your whole system would cry out, "Stop doing this, it's mad".'* Gradually, men learned to select more externally-directed strategies to manage such states. Adam realised: *'I needed to do things that took me out of myself... Better to go and see a friend, or play some music.'* Similarly, after learning from painful experience – trying to meditate while depressed – Walter found more effective ways of managing low moods, as noted in the last chapter. Being able to make such judgements is indicative of a high-level meta-coping ability.

Finally, we end this chapter by noting that narratives of control and choice were not restricted to reacting to negativity. In a more encompassing way, these skills extend to making positive choices in general with regard to wellbeing. For example, men described trying to choose activities which could enhance wellbeing, like exercising, and resist less helpful activities, like drinking. Many men discussed trying to leave behavioural patterns behind, and take on new ones. Efforts to abstain from alcohol are a prime example of men's progress here. Since taking up meditation, many men had tried to curtail their drinking, and some even abstained completely. There may have been various motives for desiring abstinence, such as health concerns. However, most men framed their abstinence efforts as linked to their engagement with meditation. For example, some said they had become inclined to stop drinking because it interfered with their ability to meditate – it affected their concentration in meditation, or in practical terms, made it hard to get up for practice. In this way, many experienced a conflict between drinking and meditating, and more broadly, between the life they had been living and the one they were drawn to. As such, trying to reduce this conflict by picking 'one or the other' was one inducement towards giving up.

Mindfulness was having an integrating effect...then I'd get drunk and it would fall apart again. I realised, 'Get drunk, or lead a life where things start to integrate'....That felt much more pleasant, [so] I found it very easy to give up. (Sam)

Other men linked their abstinence efforts to their interest in Buddhism, and its promotion of an ethical framework of 'precepts', including refraining from 'intoxication'. Here, committed Buddhists had taken vows of adherence; others were more relaxed, seeing them as idealised behaviours to be selectively pursued. Nonetheless, many men felt these were ideals worth aiming for. For William, in contrast to Christian discourses around sin he'd been brought up with (*'You feel utterly horrible'*), the precepts were helpful guidelines: *'It's a more subtle, sophisticated way of thinking...a framework for thinking about everyday life.'* Here we can see that men's engagement with wellbeing was positively influenced by the wider context in which they practised. As noted in Chapter 4, it is important not to view men's involvement with meditation in decontextualised terms. For many men, meditation was situated within a broader framework of ideas and practices – generally influenced by Buddhism – that also served to promote wellbeing.

Moreover, in considering this wider context, it is important not simply to think in abstract terms about Buddhism as a system of ideas and practices. Rather, for many men, Buddhism was experienced as a *social* phenomenon, concretely embodied in a meditation community. Most men regularly attended a meditation/Buddhist centre to meditate, where they interacted with other meditators. A helpful way of regarding these places is through Lave and Wenger's (1991) notion of communities of practice (CoP). CoP are 'people who come together around mutual engagement in an endeavour', and the practices which 'emerge in the course of this' (Eckert & McConnell-Ginet, 1992, p. 464). Crucially, as identified in Chapter 1, CoP promote local systems of hegemonic norms. Normally CoP are identified as upholding traditional forms of hegemony (Parker, 2006). Strikingly however, in the case of meditation centres an alternative 'local' system of hegemonic norms prevailed, including abstinence. In contrast to traditional hegemonic forms, which tend to uphold norms that are detrimental to wellbeing (e.g., *promoting* alcohol use), this alternative hegemonic system was positively conducive to wellbeing. Thus, men were supported in their abstinence efforts by a supportive community around meditation. For example, having spent years involved with one such community, Adam described how he had become distanced from the alcohol culture of the wider society.

> *I might have a drink, but it's very occasional. It's just not part of my life...In fact I feel a bit lost if I go in a pub now, it's just not my natural social environment.* (Adam)

As such, men's efforts to make positive behavioural choices around wellbeing depended to some extent on supportive social conditions that encouraged such efforts. (Men unconnected to meditation CoP reported more of a struggle in trying to alter their habits.) Nevertheless, the enhanced sense of control men enjoyed as a result of meditating meant they personally felt inclined and empowered to make such changes. In fact, the very decision to regularly attend a meditation group that supported one's efforts to change is indicative of enhanced emotional management skills. That is, identifying such groups as a positive resource in the pursuit of wellbeing, and then making a commitment to participate, itself reflects an example of men strategically managing their emotions. Such links between meditation and health behaviours are striking. Alcohol abuse among men is recognised as a problem, with men accounting for two thirds of alcohol deaths (ONS, 2012a). Indeed, concerns around men's alcohol use have led to 'calls to action' to encourage healthier behaviours (Courtenay, 1998). However, while various interventions have been implemented, a ten-year review concluded little progress had been made in reducing men's drinking (Robertson & Williamson, 2005). Thus, the possibility that emotional management skills inculcated by meditation can promote health behaviours like abstinence among men is striking. Andrew summed it up:

> *[Through meditation, I have] more choice to act and behave in certain ways. I can make lifestyle choices which have an impact on your health, and I find my habits that lead me away from well-being, they're less sticky, less reactive, less impulsive.*

Summary

In the last chapter, we saw that meditation could be viewed primarily as a way of developing attention/awareness skills. In the present chapter, we saw that these skills were conducive to wellbeing. In particular, by learning to attend to their inner world, men cultivated the four EI skills elucidated by Mayer and Salovey's (1997) model: emotional awareness; emotional generation of thought; emotional understanding; and the strategic management of emotions. In various ways, these skills then allowed men to engage constructively with wellbeing, in its various dimensions. This included dealing with negative thoughts and feelings, engendering 'positive' states of mind, and fostering the social aspects of wellbeing, such as interacting skilfully with others. The narratives in this area are all the more striking given men's stories of their life before meditation, where they struggled to cope with negativity, were unclear about how to promote positive states of mind, and often found themselves disconnected from other people. Thus, in a multitude of ways, meditation was an effective vehicle for these men to overcome the burden of traditional masculinity that they had grown up with, helping them to find a clearer and surer path to wellbeing.

6
Conclusions and Recommendations

It's like there's no way back, for better or worse. What a trip! Nobody told us before we embarked on this [what it would be like]! There were moments in my life, I've said, 'Shit, I should've taken [an easy life, i.e., not become a meditator]', but deep down, absolutely no hesitation, I would take it again. (Ross)

In this final chapter we draw together the findings from the previous chapters into an overall summary. This summary takes the form of nine 'lessons' that are intended to be of use to health professionals working with men, and indeed to all those with vested interest in the wellbeing of men (including, of course, men themselves). Within these lessons are recommendations that may be followed, such as practical meditation activities and ways to promote meditation engagement. The first three lessons emphasise the need for men to take up an activity like meditation: (1) under social pressure, men learn to disconnect from emotions; moreover (2) men suffer from this disconnection, and from masculinity generally; however (3) men can change, with encouragement. The next four lessons describe the value of meditation practice vis-à-vis wellbeing, showing men can learn to: (4) develop emotional awareness; (5) generate positive emotions; (6) cultivate emotional understanding; and (7) strategically manage their emotions. Finally, the last two lessons concern the maintenance of a viable practice, showing that: (8) men may struggle to maintain one and thus (9) may need the encouragement and support of others in maintaining a practice. Together, these lessons will help men in the potentially tricky but ultimately rewarding task of developing and sustaining a practice that has the great potential to enhance their wellbeing.

Lesson 1: Under social pressure, men learn to disconnect from emotions

The first lesson concerns men's emotional 'response style' – in Nolen-Hoeksema's (1987) terminology – i.e., how they habitually experience and engage with emotions. It is common to find assertions in the literature, and societal discourse generally, that males are emotionally inarticulate, stunted, or otherwise deficient. Thus, their response style is often described as one of 'restrictive emotionality', featuring emotional denial, suppression or disconnection. Clinically, the 'inability to recognize or verbalize emotions' is referred to as alexithymia (Honkalampi et al., 2000, p. 99). The association of such inability with the masculine gender has given rise to the concept of 'normative male alexithymia' (Levant, 1998). In terms of the findings here, the first point is that participants' lives prior to meditation, from adolescence onwards, were indeed coloured by such characteristic patterns of restrictive emotionality.

However, the second point to note relates to the qualifying phrase in the previous sentence, i.e., 'from adolescence onwards'. Participants were eloquently insistent that this 'restrictive' emotional style had been impressed, even forced, upon them as they navigated the difficult waters of early adolescence. Displays of emotionality and affection that were overlooked or tolerated in childhood were drummed out of most participants with the message that 'boys don't cry'. This accords with the observations of other scholars, who have identified how childhood socialisation pressures curtail the emotional expressiveness of boys (Chaplin et al., 2005), including via punitive measures like shaming from peers and family members (Mejía, 2005). This coercive process speaks to the heart of a debate around the genesis of gendered characteristics: are these inevitable products of biological characteristics of each sex, or are they behaviours encouraged by contingent socialisation pressures of our current society?

In the present study, the findings weigh heavily in favour of the latter view. Moreover, it is striking to note an especially sensitive period during early adolescence, often around age 13, when gendered norms take particular effect. There are parallels here with a study by Mac an Ghaill and Haywood (2012), who found adolescent boys awkwardly straddling a 'feminized childhood' (e.g., where emotionality was permitted) and a 'masculinized adulthood' (where it was not permitted). Similarly, in the present study, early adolescence constituted a threshold, involving a *sudden* crossing over into adulthood, on entering secondary school perhaps. At this threshold, boys were exhorted to disavow emotionality and so 'be a man'.

Thus, this first lesson cautions against essentialist or fatalistic judgements regarding any apparent emotional capabilities of males: these are learned behaviours, and are not inevitable. In terms of recommendations arising from this lesson – each lesson features practical ideas for capitalising on the findings in the book – the results urge us to pay special attention to the critical threshold period in adolescence. This seems to be a pivotal juncture where gendered behaviours, even if learned earlier in childhood, assume particular prominence as young boys feel compelled to enact an explicit model of manhood. Since schooling takes up a significant portion of adolescent boys' time, the role of educational establishments in either upholding or challenging gendered expectations is key. Indeed, the complicity of such establishments in upholding hegemonic values has been called 'poisonous pedagogy' (Kenway & Fitzclarence, 1997). Thus, helping schools to promote alternative models of masculinity may be useful in preventing boys embracing a learned restrictive emotionality. This point will be returned to below under Lesson 3.

Lesson 2: Men suffer from emotional disconnection, and masculinity generally

The reason the first lesson is so important is that restrictive emotionality had consequences for wellbeing. In learning to be tough and to disconnect from their emotions, participants developed a problematic relationship with their 'interiority', accruing a range of deleterious consequences as a result. In particular, men learned that emotions, especially ones expressing vulnerability or caring, were 'inappropriate'. While this did not mean that such emotions were not experienced – they were, indeed often forcefully – participants learned to disown or detach from these. From a psychoanalytic perspective, these were dis-identified with and repressed. There were various deleterious consequences of this disconnection: a fractured sense of identity; an inner conflict between acceptable and unacceptable aspects of their being; and, as shifting social settings required participants to disavow different aspects of themselves, a more disorienting sense of fragmentation and 'multiphrenia' (Gergen, 2001).

Thus, most men had a problematic, disconnected relationship with their interiority. Such disconnection was even more of an issue in the face of negative emotions. In these instances, learned restrictive emotionality was connected to mental health issues. As outlined in Chapter 2, Addis (2008) proposed a number of frameworks connecting masculine response styles to distress and depression. These frameworks were corroborated in the narratives. As per the masked depression framework (Cochran & Rabinowitz, 2000), some participants did recall experiencing depression as defined by generic diagnostic criteria, like low mood, but at the time had been unable to recognise it in themselves (due to restrictive emotionality). Thus their condition was 'masked' from themselves. Moreover, even if they did recognise their own distress, other masculine norms around stoicism meant that they were reluctant to reveal this to others or seek help, thus also masking it from those around.

Conversely, as per the masculine depression framework, some men did appear to experience a 'phenotypic variant of prototypic depression' (Addis, 2008, p. 159). In this case, distress was expressed in the form of 'externalising' behaviours, including anger, alcohol abuse and suicidality. These seemed to be a consequence of men's disconnection from their interiority, and subsequent inability to successfully manage their emotions. This inability, also known as 'affect dysregulation', has been identified as a 'transdiagnostic' factor underlying diverse mental health conditions (Aldao et al., 2010). In the case of men here, dysregulation meant they were unable to moderate their negative feelings, which generated consequent feelings of frustration and anger. However, it would be a mistake to simply see externalising behaviours as men 'lashing out' unconsciously. Some such behaviours can be understood as maladaptive attempts to haphazardly manage their feelings, including self-medication through alcohol (as a way of 'blunting' feelings), and even suicidality (as a way of 'stopping' their inner turmoil).

Given the association between traditional masculine norms (e.g., toughness) and emotional disconnection, and between such disconnection and mental health issues, one might say that traditional masculinity is a 'risk factor' for mental health issues. This aligns with a wider popular discourse that masculinity is a risk factor for health generally (Gough, 2006), since masculinity is linked to health risk behaviours, including alcohol use, poor diet and risk-taking (Courtenay, 2000). Traditional masculine norms also adversely affected wellbeing in other ways too, which then intersected with issues arising from affect dysregulation. For example, norms around independence and invulnerability encouraged participants to adopt a 'lone man' stance. Adapting Bakan's (1966) terminology, men here became 'hyperagentic'. However, especially problematic was the finding that men were most likely to enact this stance when they were in distress, i.e., at the times when they might have benefitted most from others' help. Thus they had less access to social networks that could have supported them in such difficult times, an isolation that is commonly observed in men (Davidson, 2004).

In terms of recommendations arising here, I echo exhortations by Oliffe and Phillips (2008) in calling for more sensitivity – from health professionals, and society generally – in dealing with distress and mental health issues in men. It is argued that health professionals may have tendencies to overlook depression in men. For example, aspects of 'masculine depression', such as anger attacks, may be unlikely to be revealed in clinical interviews (Winkler et al., 2006). Even if externalising behaviours are uncovered in such situations, clinicians may hone in on the presenting symptoms, like alcohol abuse, and overlook the underlying distress (Rabinowitz & Cochran, 2008). Thus, greater sensitivity to men's distress, and of the ways in which men conspire to conceal or otherwise fail to manage this, is needed. In terms of men themselves, we can agree with Kilmartin (2005, p. 97) that they should be educated to 'resist the cultural pressure to be masculine', thus hopefully lessening the likelihood of experiencing distress related to masculinity.

Lesson 3: Men can change, with encouragement

To the extent that men here 'suffered' due to masculinity, as outlined in Lesson 2, the findings concur with the 'masculinity as risk-factor' discourse identified by Gough (2006). However, as Addis (2008) himself recognised in outlining his models linking masculinity to depression and distress, his models did not account for recent constructionist theorising acknowledging variation in men and masculinities. My interviews account for just that, showing not only that some men can and do engage constructively with their wellbeing, but more importantly, that men can *change*. That is, as seen in Lessons 1 and 2, most men here reported succumbing to masculine norms around toughness to some extent. Thus, many had difficulties engaging with their emotions, with subsequent implications for mental health. However, all men here learned to change and adopt behaviours more conducive to wellbeing, in this case, taking up meditation.

Consequently, the findings belie the fatalistic, essentialist forms of discourse – common in the literature on gender, and within society at large – that construct men as inevitably and inextricably emotionally inarticulate. I have previously suggested that this more 'hopeful' perspective on men and masculinity could be termed 'critical positive masculinity' (Lomas, 2013). The prefix 'positive' serves to align this with the positive psychology movement, which is concerned with studying and helping people to be 'at their best' (Seligman et al., 2005). However, there is an existing 'positive masculinity' paradigm which strives to find virtue in 'traditional' male qualities, including courage and strength (Kiselica & Englar-Carlson, 2010). In contrast, the approach detailed in this book has been to explore how men might challenge or redefine traditional masculinity. Thus the prefix 'critical' serves to reflect the 'critical studies on men' paradigm, which seeks to 'problematise' and challenge the status quo around gender (Hearn, 1997).

The crucial questions for the purposes of this third lesson are, how did this change occur, and what lessons can be learned in terms of encouraging other men to make similar changes? The key route into answering these is to note that there was variation in how soon, how easily, and for what reasons different men turned to meditation. A small minority sought out a different way of being in early adulthood, and embraced meditation easily. Some men turned to meditation slightly later in life as a way of better managing stress/distress. Others became dissatisfied with life and embarked on a difficult process of existential questioning, leading eventually to meditation. Finally, about half of men only turned to meditation following a crisis, such as an emotional breakdown.

There are two main points to mention regarding the differences between these various groups of men. First, the sooner men turned to meditation, the better their prognosis vis-à-vis mental health and general wellbeing: the minority who found meditation in early adulthood said it helped them weather the inevitable storms of life and moderate its stresses; in contrast, the last group depicted the most serious issues, including mental health problems, which they invariably failed to deal with constructively. The second point is the most instructive for the purposes of our discussion here, and deals with *why* some men turned to meditation earlier and with greater ease than others. In particular, those who found meditation sooner were those men who had the confidence and/or encouragement to resist or redefine traditional masculine norms. This beneficent independence generally depended upon men having been raised within a supportive family environment that encouraged them to 'go their own way'.

Thus, we can draw on these findings to make various recommendations. First, the sooner in life males can be encouraged to engage with their emotions, for example through meditation, the better. In this respect, it is encouraging to note that there are a number of programmes for taking meditation into schools (e.g., Broderick & Metz, 2009; Schonert-Reichl & Lawlor, 2010). These programmes acknowledge the need to adapt meditation for use with a younger age group, for instance making the sessions shorter, less cognitively demanding, and more 'fun'. However, one flaw with such programmes is that they appear to make no provision for gender considerations. In particular, they do not take into account the possibility that activities such as meditation may run counter to masculine norms that encourage boys to be tough. Thus, as beneficial as such programmes may be, unless gender-based countervailing social pressures are addressed, boys may be reluctant to take part in the first place.

So, a second recommendation is to explicitly factor gender into these programmes, designing them to counter prohibitive masculinity expectations. However, while it may be desirable to teach boys to 'resist' such expectations, this may be unrealistic. A more attainable route may be to help boys re-interpret these in beneficent ways instead. For example, norms around independence are seen as discouraging men from seeking help for health problems. However, Noone and Stephens (2008) found some men were skilfully able to re-interpret help-seeking as an *example* of independence (e.g., resisting expectations). Thus, rather than just instructing boys not to be tough, a more prosperous route may be to cast the emotional control developed through meditation as an example of toughness, perhaps by associating meditation with exemplars of toughness, like martial artists. In this way, working with the stream of masculine expectations, but recasting these in positive ways, boys may find it easier to try meditation without misgivings or resistance.

Lesson 4: Men can develop emotional awareness

It is all very well appealing to men to change and engage with their emotions. However, what is needed are concrete, practical activities to actually help them achieve this (otherwise such exhortations are liable to be as ineffectual as simply telling people with depression to 'cheer up'; if they knew how, the advice would be unnecessary). Herein lay the value of meditation: a simple technique – simple to comprehend, if not necessarily to execute – for men to learn the skills they were lacking. In Chapter 4 we saw that the term 'meditation' covered a wide variety of different methods. Nevertheless, it was established that learning how to regulate one's attention was the 'central commonality' across the divergent methods (Cahn & Polich, 2006, p. 180). Thus, we can view meditation as primarily a method for developing attention and awareness (cognisant of the subtle differences between these two phenomena). Speaking more poetically, we might describe meditation as an introspective practice that allows people to explore their 'inner world'. Moreover, cultivating such awareness was just the first step in a broader process of men developing the four branches of EI (Mayer & Salovey, 1997), as will be explored in this chapter (with Lessons 4 to 7 each focusing on one particular branch, beginning here with the first branch, awareness).

Meditation has been established as a beneficial practice for both clinical and non-clinical populations, reducing mental health issues and enhancing wellbeing (Mars & Abbey, 2010). What is unique about the findings reported in this book is the particular value of meditation for *men* specifically. Lessons 1 and 2 show how men often become emotionally disconnected due to acquiescing to masculine norms. In this context, meditation was the corrective they needed to re-connect emotionally and begin to redress their learned emotional deficiencies. Through meditation, men took tentative steps to explore their interiority. This task could be difficult at times, especially at first. Men found it difficult to interiorise their attention, this being an unfamiliar activity, and had challenges remaining attentive. More unsettling, men encountered troubling thoughts and feelings which they had previously disconnected from (often precisely because such qualia were painful). Nevertheless, all participants valued the process of developing emotional awareness and becoming 're-acquainted' with themselves.

In terms of specific meditation practices, men undertook a diverse range. Following Mikulas (1990), these practices can be distinguished according to four parameters. First, behaviours of mind, where scholars differentiate between two types of attention/awareness: focused attention (FA) and open monitoring (OM), the latter more commonly referred to as mindfulness. Second, focus: meditation practices can take a range of stimuli as their object, both external (e.g., a shrine) and internal (e.g., thoughts and feelings); additionally, OM practices are intended to be 'un-focused', i.e., not fixed on a particular object. Third, attitude: practitioners are encouraged to imbue their attention/awareness with positive attitudinal qualities, ranging from the relatively neutral (e.g., acceptance), to more strongly qualified (e.g., compassion), even up to stances of reverence. Finally, form: meditation can be practised in various physical postures, including moving (e.g., yoga or walking), lying down, and most commonly, sitting.

While recognising the diversity of practices however, there was one basic core practice that served as most participants' introduction to meditation: mindfulness. A prominent definition of mindfulness is the 'awareness that arises through paying attention on purpose, in the present moment, and nonjudgementally to the unfolding of experience moment by moment' (Kabat-Zinn, 2003, p. 145). Following Kabat-Zinn's (1982) pioneering MBSR programme, mindfulness has become the pre-eminent focus of academic and clinical research on meditation (Brown et al., 2007). In terms of engendering this sought-after state in practi-tioners, a wide range of techniques has been identified. Perhaps the most common of these – within the narratives here, and in meditation liter-ature more generally – is the 'mindfulness of breathing'. Men described this as a simple introductory technique that enabled them to begin to develop their emotional awareness.

In the interest of offering practical recommendations to readers who may be working with men (or to men themselves reading this), this concluding chapter offers basic instructions for various meditation prac-tices, beginning in this lesson with the mindfulness of breathing. (As with the guidance offered in subsequent lessons, these instructions are but one variant of the practices; other sources may differ in their advice, and readers should in any case feel free to adapt these recommenda-tions to their needs and sensibilities.) The mindfulness of breathing is often conducted in five stages. The title is actually a misnomer. The prac-tice begins with focused attention on the breath – FA rather than OM – which does not constitute mindfulness proper. 'Genuine' mindfulness only begins in the last stage of the practice, once attention has been sta-bilised through FA, which helps stop the mind 'wandering' during OM (Chiesa et al., 2011). The following instructions may be spoken aloud or otherwise given to participants. As with instructions for other practices below, the duration is flexible. However, for beginners it is worth aiming for at least 15 minutes in total (thus each of the five stages should last at least a few minutes).

- Sitting quietly and comfortably, close your eyes, and take a few moments to feel your breath slowing down.
- This practice has five stages. . . . So, beginning with Stage 1.
- As you breathe in and out, quietly say 'one' at the end of the out-breath.
- As you breathe in and out again, quietly say 'two' at the end of the out-breath.
- In this way, continue counting until you have reached ten, then begin again at one.

- If your mind drifts off before you reach ten, as soon as you notice it has done so, gently bring your attention back to the breath, beginning your count again at one.

- Now in Stage 2, continue counting your breaths, with each in-and-out breath together being one number.
- This time though, instead of saying the number at the end of the out-breath, say it at the beginning of the in-breath.

- Now in Stage 3, stop counting, and just focus on the sensation of breathing.
- Pay particular attention to your nostrils, and the way the breath feels cool coming in through the tip of your nose, and warmer as it passes out again.

- Now in Stage 4, again refraining from counting, move your attention to your stomach.
- Pay particular attention to your diaphragm, and the way this gently moves out and down as you breathe in, and in and up as you breathe out.

- Now in this final stage, let go of your focus on your breath.
- Instead, just sit and allow yourself to be aware of any thoughts, feelings or sensations that are arising in your mind and your body.
- Whatever arises, try not to dwell on it or give it too much attention – simply note its presence.
- Imagine that your mind is the clear blue sky, and thoughts and feelings are just clouds passing through; the sky is not affected by their presence – they pass through and don't leave a mark.
- In the same way, thoughts and feelings pass through your awareness, but your awareness is separate from these, and is unchanged by them.
- Sitting peacefully, stay in this mindful state for as long as you are comfortable.
- Then relax your awareness, sit quietly for a few breaths, and then slowly open your eyes, and finish.

Finally, it is important to note that, ideally, practitioners engage in mindfulness meditation practices with the aim of remaining mindful *outside* of such practices. Men emphasised the idea that meditation should not be an escapist activity, circumscribed from the rest of life – although they admitted such escapism did sometimes happen. Rather, they endeavoured to maintain qualities and states of mind generated in meditation, like mindfulness, throughout their other daily activities. Similarly, this aim is central to mindfulness interventions, like MBSR (Kabat-Zinn, 2003), which augment their taught sessions with homework activities. Building on mindfulness techniques taught during the sessions, participants are exhorted to attempt to undertake daily activities in a mindful way. Participants are usually encouraged to begin by just trying this for one activity per day (e.g., the morning shower), before extending this to other activities. As such, readers of this book teaching mindfulness to others, or indeed readers themselves, might similarly seek to encourage this kind of everyday 'meditation-in-action' (Bruce & Davies, 2005).

Lesson 5: Men can generate positive emotions

As noted in Lesson 4, enhanced awareness *per se* had the potential to be problematic: turning inwards in meditation, men sometimes became aware of troubling qualia, such as negative self-referential thoughts, which could be upsetting. As emphasised by meditation scholars, participants found it important to augment their awareness with an 'openhearted, friendly' and 'affectionate, compassionate quality' (Kabat-Zinn, 2003, p. 145). Unfortunately, men often had difficulty generating these requisite qualities, a finding often overlooked in the meditation literature. Thankfully, many participants came across a specific practice explicitly designed to inculcate feelings of compassion, the *'metta bhavana'* (translated as 'the practice of loving kindness'). This practice, operationalised in the literature as 'loving-kindness meditation' (LKM), is effective in reducing mental illness and distress, and enhancing wellbeing, in both clinical (Johnson et al., 2009) and non-clinical populations (Fredrickson et al., 2008).

Similarly, most men here greatly valued the practice. Some specifically highlighted the fact that it 'allowed' them to cultivate and experience caring qualities which they had previously learned to view as contrary to masculine ideals and 'inappropriate' for men. In augmenting their burgeoning attention skills with the ability to generate positive emotions with which to suffuse this attention, we discern a pattern. In particular, the development of cognitive skills through meditation followed something of a sequence, one which can be broadly mapped onto Mayer and Salovey's (1997) hierarchical model of EI. Their model features four branches. The lower two branches, collectively labelled as experiential

EI, are 'emotional awareness and expression', and the 'emotional facilitation of thought' ('ability to generate emotions'; Day & Carroll, 2004, p. 1444). These two branches are represented here in Lessons 4 and 5 respectively. (The higher two branches, together referred to as strategic EI, are the ability to 'understand emotional patterns' and the 'strategic management of emotions'. These are covered in Lessons 6 and 7.)

The *metta bhavana* (or LKM in psychological terminology) is usually constructed as a five-stage process, although this structure admits variations (Salzberg, 2004). First, practitioners are encouraged to generate feelings of *metta* for themselves. The key here is that practitioners see themselves as ordinary people, beset by human failings and troubles, who are nonetheless just trying their best to find some happiness in this life. As they sit to meditate, they may try to reflect on this viewpoint, while rehearsing self-affirmative statements. These statements can be anchored to the act of breathing, just as the mindfulness of breathing practice did with ascending numbers. Here, instead of enumerating the influx and efflux of respiration, in- and out-breaths can be vehicles for various affirmative statements (see below). The remaining four stages take the same process, except switching the focus from the practitioner themselves to various other people: a close friend or family member; a 'neutral' person; an antagonist (someone they dislike or with whom they have a difficult relationship); and 'people in general'. In terms of teaching the practice, the following instructions may be spoken aloud or otherwise given to participants. Let the participant continue in each stage for at least two to three minutes (longer if possible), before moving them on to the next stage.

- Sitting quietly and comfortably, close your eyes, and take a few moments to feel your breath slowing down.
- In this first stage, reflect on the fact that you are a normal person, suffering from ordinary human failings, who is nevertheless trying to find some happiness in life.
- As you breathe in, say softly, 'May I be happy.'
- As you breathe out, say softly, 'May I be well.'
- As you breathe in, say softly, 'May I be free from suffering.'
- As you breathe out, say softly, 'May I be free.'
- Continue breathing, repeating these phrases on the in- and out-breaths.

- Now bring to mind a person you feel close to, perhaps a friend or family member.

- Reflect on the fact that, just like you, they are a normal person, suffering from ordinary human failings, who is nevertheless trying to find some happiness in life.
- Repeat the same phrases as before, substituting 'you' for 'I': 'May you be happy' (breathing in); 'May you be well' (breathing out); 'May you be free from suffering' (breathing in); 'May you be free' (breathing out).

- Now bring to mind a person for whom you have no strong feelings, perhaps someone you encounter regularly, like a local shopkeeper, but rarely give a thought to.
- Reflect on the fact that, just like you, they are a normal human being, suffering from ordinary human failings, who is nevertheless trying to get by and find some happiness in their life.
- Repeat the same phrases as the previous stage, keeping with 'you' (e.g., 'May you be happy').

- Now bring to mind a person who you dislike, or find difficult or challenging.
- Reflect on the fact that, just like you, they are a normal person, suffering from ordinary human failings, who is nevertheless trying to find some happiness in life.
- Repeat the same phrases as the previous stage, keeping with 'you' (e.g., 'May you be happy').

- Now bring to mind all the people you know personally.
- Reflect on the fact that, just like you, they are normal people, suffering from ordinary human failings, who are nevertheless trying to find some happiness in life.
- Repeat the same phrases as the previous stage, keeping with 'you' (e.g., 'May you be happy').
- Continue breathing, repeating these phrases on the in- and out-breaths.
- [After a minute] Now extend your focus to everyone in your community.
- [After a minute] Now extend your focus to everyone in your home country.
- [After a minute] Now extend your focus to everyone in the world.

Another practice for generating compassion is one of 'giving and taking', of which there are numerous variants (Gyatso, 2009). In subtly different ways, these variants have practitioners actively imagining taking on the sufferings of others, and giving positive emotions in return. As with the self-affirmative statements in the *metta bhavana*, these practices use a focus on the breath as a vehicle for generating this interchange: the inward and outward currents of air are linked imaginatively to ideas of taking and giving respectively. For example, a participant might be encouraged to bring to mind a person close to them who is suffering under some hardship. On each in-breath, the participant might imagine 'drawing in' this person's suffering into themselves, perhaps visualised in the form of a plume of noxious smoke. The participant may then picture this smoke being dissipated in their 'heart' by the power of their affection. Then, on the out-breath, the participant imagines emanating positive feelings towards the person in question, visualised in the form of a beam of white light, issuing forth from their own heart and enveloping the other person. In terms of teaching the practice, this cyclical visualisation process of giving (happiness) and taking (suffering) can be summarised with the following instructions, which can be spoken aloud or otherwise given to participants.

- Sitting quietly and comfortably, close your eyes, and take a few moments to feel your breath slowing down.
- Bring to mind a person, to whom you are close, who has recently suffered some trouble or hardship.
- Spend a few moments thinking about their suffering, and how you would like to relieve them of this if possible.
- Visualise their suffering as a cloud of noxious black smoke, enveloping them.
- Breathing in, imagine that you are drawing in this smoke through your nostrils.
- As you do, softly say, 'May I take away your troubles.'
- At the still-point at the end of the in-breath, imagine this black smoke being dissolved in your heart by the force of your affection for this person.
- Visualise this affection as a clear, white light.
- Breathing out, imagine that you are emanating this white light, which bathes the person in a radiant cloud of your affection.
- As you do, softly say, 'May I give you happiness.'
- Repeat this process, 'taking in' suffering on each in-breath, and 'giving out' happiness on each out-breath.
- Continue for as long as you feel comfortable, ideally for no less than five minutes.

Lesson 6: Men can cultivate emotional understanding

Through long-term regular meditation practice, men began to cultivate an understanding of their emotional dynamics. Thus, continuing the sequence of EI skill development, having initially learned simply to attend to their emotions, and then to generate emotions, men began developing the third branch of EI – emotional understanding. The types of insights men shared in their narratives were diverse, complex and sophisticated. Together these insights offer a robust rebuttal to the notion of men as inevitably emotionally inarticulate. Moreover, that these men had previously felt they had been emotionally stunted or disconnected, as per Lessons 1 and 2, is evidence that men can change and develop their emotional capabilities. Once again, this is an endorsement for the more hopeful perspective on men underpinning the proposed 'critical positive masculinity' paradigm.

So, men offered a wide range of emotional insights. Some of these were more personal, and are not necessarily generalisable. For example, some participants noted a tendency to repeat particular ruminative self-critical thought patterns. Echoing cognitive theories of depression (e.g., Teasdale, 1988), they now understood that becoming 'drawn in' to these ruminations had the potential to precipitate a descent into low moods, and even bouts of depression. Through meditation, men learned to identify these habitual mental patterns, enabling them to recognise these as just an unfortunate quirk of their mental conditioning. Such recognition enabled men to 'decentre' from these patterns – observing and hence disregarding them in a detached way as ephemeral mental phenomena, rather than accurate statements about the self that were true and needed to be believed.

Other insights were more generic – though no less powerful – and may be relevant to the majority of readers. I shall briefly note two of the most common. First, the ephemeral nature of mental patterns, as noted above, was generalised by many participants to all subjective phenomena. The notion that all thoughts, feelings and sensations are fleeting and temporary is a central Buddhist teaching (Kumar, 2002), one to which most men assented. This insight is captured poetically by the phrase, 'This too will pass.' This notion helped men 'sit with' negative qualia in meditation, duly reassured that their discomfort would be temporary. A second common insight was that thoughts and emotions are somatised – i.e., have physical components that can be viscerally felt in the body. Men were then able to profitably combine these two insights in meditation to relieve negative emotions. That is, when distressed, rather than ruminating on the causes of their dysphoria, men were able to focus on the physical manifestation of this distress and observe it changing and dissipating.

These two insights were not the result of a specific meditation practice. Rather, they tended to be won through repeated engagement with various generic practices, like mindfulness, over an extended period of time. However, we are at liberty here to construct a practice that does capture the insights expressed by participants in a form that may engender these insights in others. Thus, the following instructions are not taken from an existent practice, but are an attempt at formulating a new practice. (The novelty of these instructions should not deter people from attempting it. Indeed, readers should be encouraged to develop their own novel practices based on their own psychological theories and insights. Once it is appreciated that meditation is a broad term for deploying attention in skilful ways, there are no necessary limits to the ways in which people can be taught to deploy this attention for their benefit.) The following instructions are designed to be spoken or otherwise given to practitioners who may be currently experiencing distress or dysphoria.

- Sitting quietly and comfortably, close your eyes, and take a few moments to feel your breath slowing down.
- As you sit, allow yourself to acknowledge any negativity you may be feeling.
- As you acknowledge this, rather than trying to think about your suffering, or dwelling on its origins and trying to work out solutions, see if you can *feel* it in your body.
- Perhaps you're anxious – maybe this can be felt as a nervous energy in your chest?
- Or perhaps you're feeling sad – maybe this is experienced as dull heaviness in your stomach?
- Whatever your emotion, try to explore the way it is physically expressing itself as a sensation in your body.
- Having found the physical location of your emotion, turn towards this sensation with a kind, curious, forgiving kind of awareness.
- You are not trying to change, amplify or get rid of the sensation. You are simply letting it be, and observing how it feels.
- Now try to describe the sensation – if it were a colour, what colour would it be; if it were a shape, what shape would it be?

- As you observe the sensation with a kindly curiosity, perhaps you notice it changing, taking on a different form, maybe shrinking in size.
- Perhaps the change is small, almost imperceptible, but nevertheless it is there.
- As you notice this change, reflect on the idea that feelings and sensations are not solid objects, existing permanently through space and time, but are ever changing and evolving.
- As you reflect on this idea, say the phrase, 'This too will pass.'
- As you continue to breathe in and out, while staying focused on the sensations in your body, softly repeat this phrase with each out-breath.
- Continue for as long as you are comfortable doing so.
- Then bring your attention up out of the body, sit quietly for a few breaths, and then slowly open your eyes, and finish.

Lesson 7: Men can strategically manage their emotions

The previous three lessons suggested that, through meditation, in a more or less sequential fashion, men developed the first three EI branches: emotional awareness, the ability to generate emotions, and emotional understanding. The development of these capacities then culminated in the fourth branch: strategic emotional management. If the first three branches were to be regarded as adaptive coping responses, this fourth branch might be viewed as a 'meta-coping' ability (Carver & Scheier, 1998). That is, bringing awareness to bear upon negative emotions, or generating positive emotions, were effective coping responses for distress, as well as being productive routes to wellbeing generally. However, meta-coping ability refers to a higher-level skill in which people are reflexively aware of a range of different potential responses (rather than automatically engaging a particular response). They are then able to skilfully select from these as appropriate to meet the particular demands of the situation. So, while various meditation practices, and resultant qualities and skills, were conducive to wellbeing, with experience, men became better able to judge *which* practice to deploy in order to achieve a desired outcome.

Moreover, this strategic meta-coping capacity meant men became skilled at managing their emotions through responses *other* than meditation. That is, while meditation was conducive to wellbeing, the emotional understanding it engendered meant participants also became good at engaging in other activities which could generate wellbeing. For example, men understood that wellbeing was also promoted by such activities as eating a healthy diet, refraining from alcohol/drugs, taking regular exercise, cultivating friendships, and being part of a community. Before taking up meditation, men were less likely to engage in activities such as these, partly because they are regarded as contrary to the prescriptions of traditional masculinity, as outlined in Chapters 2 and 3 (Courtenay, 2000). However, through meditation, men had a better understanding of the merits of such activities. More importantly, men also developed the wherewithal, motivation and behavioural control to engage in these activities. Moreover, as part of their 'meta-coping' capacity, men became skilled at judging which behaviour best suited their emotional needs at that time. For example, at points, talking with a friend might be the optimal strategy; at a different point, exercising alone may be the better response.

Paradoxically, a vital aspect of this capacity for strategic management, acquired through meditation, is knowing when *not* to meditate. The narratives were unusual in revealing a range of potentially serious problems connected to meditation, showing meditation can be harmful under certain circumstances. Such risks are rarely noted in the literature (Irving et al., 2009). Meditating while depressed could worsen men's mood, drawing them further into rumination, since they lack the strength to decentre. (This risk is acknowledged by the originators of Mindfulness-Based Cognitive Therapy for depression, who emphasise that it is contraindicated for those *currently* depressed; Teasdale et al., 2003.) Similarly, meditation exacerbated states of strong anxiety, since it made participants more sensitive to stimuli that provoked such anxiety. More seriously, there were suggestions that certain 'advanced' meditations, like the 'Six element' practice, aimed at 'deconstructing the self', had the potential to precipitate psychotic episodes if practised incorrectly. Causality is hard to determine here; however, meditation has been found to precipitate psychosis in those with a history of the condition, and is thus contraindicated for this population (Lustyk et al., 2009).

With experience, participants became more adept at avoiding these risks. Men learned to recognise that for certain negative states of mind, an introspective response like meditation was inappropriate; better perhaps to select a behavioural strategy like exercise. Regarding the risk of severe adverse psychological reactions from advanced practices, men learned to seek expert guidance in attempting these practices, and to avail themselves of the insights of such experts in interpreting the anomalous (i.e., exceptional) experiences that could result from such practices. Thus, the intention here is not to finish these lessons on meditation on a sour note: all men strongly felt that meditation was highly valuable and rewarding; they simply emphasised that it was a potent activity, with the potential to powerfully affect one's mind, and needed to be respected as such. However, this kind of 'wisdom of experience' will be unavailable to those new to meditation. As such, for readers seeking to utilise meditation in their professional work (e.g., in psychotherapeutic practice), it is appropriate to offer a number of recommendations concerning its use:

- Practices focusing on thoughts or emotions may be inadvisable for clients in a state of anxiety or low mood; exercises focusing on breathing may be more appropriate.
- Meditation can bring people into contact with troubling thoughts/ feelings: clients may need to be supported after the meditation session in working through these.
- Men may have particular difficulties with meditation on account of prior tendencies towards restrictive emotionality; men may need assistance in recognising emotions, and cultivating positive qualities like self-compassion.
- If advising clients to try meditation in the community, do so with caution – clients may encounter difficulties in meditation, but lack the therapeutic support at the time to help them manage these.

Relating to this last point, there are also some recommendations for teachers and centres offering meditation in the community. It would be advisable for such centres/teachers to have the following protocols in place:

- Screening of participants in terms of present mental state, with a wider remit than psychiatric history (e.g., monitoring current mood).
- Those judged to be at risk (e.g., in a state of anxiety) advised to try meditation only under the guidance of a qualified clinical practitioner, or at the least be carefully monitored by the session leader.
- All participants be informed of potential risks, and be given opportunities to withdraw.
- Session leaders should make provisions for spending time after the session with any participants who may wish to discuss concerns.

• Have information and contact details for clinical and psychother-apeutic services to hand for anyone who appears to have been particularly troubled by the session.

Lesson 8: Men may struggle to maintain a practice

The four lessons above have shown meditation to be highly benefi-cial to men's wellbeing, even with the caveats about potential risks included in Lesson 7. However, as much as these benefits were noted and appreciated by participants themselves, many nevertheless struggled – at least some of the time – to maintain their practice. Despite widespread academic and clinical interest in meditation, such issues are rarely addressed in the literature, and little is known about how people engage with it in the context of their everyday lives. Most studies are based on controlled interventions of limited duration, and usually fail to assess home practice outside formal sessions (Vettese et al., 2009). If issues around practice maintenance *are* noted, it is generally only as a method-ological limitation, rather than an object of interest in its own right. The narratives here reveal a range of issues and obstacles that conspired to curtail, hinder or otherwise disrupt men's engagement with meditation. There were three main types of issues: practical, motivational and social. These can be considered in turn.

In terms of practical issues, a range of other life commitments vied with meditation for men's time, as detailed at greater length in Lomas et al. (2013). Since people generally lead busy lives, there is noth-ing remarkable about this observation. It is still pertinent however, as most research on meditation is highly decontextualised, and over-looks the sheer difficulty that many people have simply finding time to sit to practise. Moreover, while every period in history may feel particularly demanding to those living through it, men were of the opinion that our current age was especially un-conducive to pursuing a meditative lifestyle. Among the causes cited were the stress of city living, the omnipresent distractions of technology and advertising, a perilous labour market that undermined one's sense of security, and an ever-demanding work environment. Regarding those last two points, it is worth contextualising the research and noting that it occurred in the wake of the 2008 financial crash, which produced rising unem-ployment and job insecurity (Bell & Blanchflower, 2010). Readers will be familiar with the demands of this current time, and can appreci-ate the way life pressures can compromise one's best efforts to lead a better life.

With motivation, men recalled periods when their interest in, and commitment to, meditation waned, and even dissipated for a time. For some, the learning curve in which they became acquainted with the potential risks of meditation – detailed in Lesson 7 – could be especially dispiriting. Although men eventually understood that meditating while depressed was counterproductive, this insight was hard-won, the result of actually trying to meditate under such conditions and experiencing the adverse consequences. At the time, these experiences undermined belief in the value and efficacy of meditation, thus draining men's motivation. Even without adversity, men sometimes became disenchanted on the grounds that meditation was not generating the type of positive experiences they had expected it to. Many endorsed a narrative of progress, in which they believed that meditation should, and would, lead to personal development and wellbeing. Whilst this progress narrative was often borne out – men did generally feel that life was improving due to meditation – this was not always the case. Sometimes it felt that meditation was just more like hard work, plodding along for no reward. At such times too, men could feel dispirited, and question whether the activity justified the time and effort put into it.

More insidiously, there were various societal counter-pressures that discouraged men from meditating. As seen in Chapter 3, these pressures had initially put some men off meditation. This led to delays and procrastination that were only overcome when their distress reached such severity that they threw caution to the wind in the hope of a solution. Some counter-pressures related to gender specifically; others were more generic. With the former, men recalled feeling that 'spiritual' activities – which is how they and others perceived meditation – contravened traditional masculine norms around toughness and rationality (the latter of which is also regarded as a masculine norm; Ross-Smith & Kornberger, 2004). In terms of generic proscriptions, some men suggested that although meditation had become increasingly 'visible' and normalised in contemporary Western culture, it was still regarded with suspicion by many people they knew; this seemed to be a particular issue for those men of lower socio-economic status (SES). This last point will be returned to below.

This perceived societal antipathy to meditation was not simply experienced in an abstract sense. Some men were censured and even ostracised by their peers and even their family for their interest in meditation and Buddhism. In the case of peers, this was because men were transgressing traditional masculine norms (e.g., by pursuing abstinence) and departing from peer group norms. With families, some regarded Buddhism with suspicion as a 'cult', while a few Christian families were perturbed by their son eschewing the Christian faith in favour of Buddhism. In search of social support and validation for their interest in meditation, many men became involved with meditation centres, interacting with others who shared their enthusiasm. Such centres were vital in support-ing men's meditation practice, as discussed further in Lesson 9. Even with the support of these places, men still faced a sense of conflict when trying to uphold their identity as a meditator in the 'outside world'. For example, men were wary of expressing the qualities cultivated through meditation – such as compassion or relational intimacy – outside of their meditation centres as fully as they would like, for fear of hegemonic censure.

Returning to the point above about SES, hegemonic censure for engag-ing in meditation was particularly prevalent for men from lower SES backgrounds. SES was not a primary focus of the research, nor was it specifically enquired about. Nevertheless, it did emerge as a factor in the counter-pressure that many men faced that discouraged their engage-ment in meditation, as men from relatively disadvantaged backgrounds found it especially difficult to challenge hegemonic expectations. This intersection of SES and gender reflects research by Seale and Charteris-Black (2008, p. 466), who suggested that higher SES men may find it easier to fashion a 'more reflexive and critical perspective on con-ventional masculinity' as their 'greater cultural capital involves access to a wider discursive repertoire' of emotions. In contrast, as Harris (2000) also found, lower SES men here had less access to resources that help in the construction of a successful (i.e., powerful) masculine identity, such as education and employment. As such, these men were more likely to resort to aggressive 'hyperagentic' behaviours (based on strength/aggression) to assert their status as men.

Socio-economic status was not a central focus of the research in this book. However, the 'intersectionality' of masculinity and SES – the way different identity categories 'intersect' to create complexities in each particular category (Hankivsky & Christoffersen, 2008) – with regard to wellbeing needs to be a priority in terms of future research. This lesson has focused on the difficulties men faced in maintaining their practice, which was the case across different socio-economic strata. Those work-ing with men need to be cognisant of and sensitive to these difficulties. However, such difficulties may be comparatively greater for males of lower SES. Thus in terms of specific recommendations arising from this particular lesson, here the call is for more research in helping males from disadvantaged backgrounds to profit from beneficial wellbeing practices such as meditation. There are promising interventions targeted towards at-risk males, e.g., resiliency programmes (Smokowski, 1998); these can serve as models for helping bring practices like meditation to populations that may benefit most from them.

Lesson 9: Men need encouragement and support from others

This final lesson follows on from the concerns raised in Lesson 8 regarding the challenges men faced in maintaining a meditation practice, and indeed in taking up such a practice in the first place. The key point in this ninth lesson is that, for the most part, the solution to these challenges lies in men receiving encouragement and support from others. Initially, this might mean steering men towards considering the idea of meditation in the first place. If interest is stimulated, this would involve exhorting men to actually practise, for example joining a class. If men do then start, this support may lie in fanning the flames of their nascent enthusiasm, and/or quelling any incipient doubts. Once men have taken to practising, they will need help in maintaining this in the face of the challenges outlined above. Thus, this important support and encouragement will pertain to all types of challenges – practical, motivational and social.

First, as noted above, some challenges were practical, like finding time in an already busy schedule to meditate. Here we can appeal for help from others with significant roles in men's lives. For example, partners/families may support men in finding ten minutes in the morning to meditate, especially if it is appreciated that this will be time well spent (rather than an indulgent luxury). Similarly, the organisations that occupy much of males' time – schools for boys, workplaces for men – may be encouraged to afford them opportunities to practise. For example, workplaces could permit scheduled breaks for employees to practise; going further, such organisations could even offer classes themselves, structured into the working day, as indeed some are already doing (Cooper & Cartwright, 1994). For employers concerned about 'indulging' their employees in this way, they can be reassured that meditation has been found to increase workers' efficiency and productivity, thus promoting the 'bottom line' (Tischler et al., 2002). This is in addition to simply enhancing employee wellbeing, and creating a 'positive emotional climate' in the workplace, the importance and value of which is increasingly recognised by employers (Ashkanasy & Daus, 2002).

Practical challenges like finding time to practise are easily recognised and so are arguably more straightforward to address. More insidious, and therefore harder to acknowledge and rectify, are motivational and social challenges. Lesson 8 suggested that hegemonic pressures can discourage men from taking up meditation, and can cause social conflict, censure and even ostracism if men do. Given these prohibitive social pressures against men practising meditation – which in themselves represent an important finding, and have hitherto not been identified – the key question is, what can be *done* about it? We can certainly hope for a more enlightened society in which traditional masculinity norms are not so weighed against constructive engagement with wellbeing, and indeed we should agitate for such a society. However, such idealistic pan-societal change may be unrealistic in the short term. As such, we need to find more attainable solutions in the near term to help those men who do wish to embrace practices like meditation, and indeed take on new ways of being a man generally.

A potential solution lies in the narratives here. Whether by accident or design, most men found themselves becoming involved with meditation centres to some extent. These offered opportunities for men to socialise with others interested in meditation, to practise alongside them and learn in a communal way. This description actually plays down the significance of such places: these were not merely locations facilitating communal practice; their value to men was far greater. In particular, such centres functioned as communities of practice (CoP) (Lave & Wenger, 1991). The importance of these was that they provided an alternative local system of masculine hegemony to the traditional forms encountered outside them. Here, emotional expression, in-depth relationships and spiritual development were valorised. The support and encouragement of such CoP was crucial in supporting men's meditation practice, and in helping them to take on new ways of being a man more generally, such as abstinence and interpersonal intimacy.

As such, the final recommendation here is to encourage men to seek out and join such CoP, or even to form their own. There are many established meditation centres in the UK, and of course worldwide. Information about such centres is easily found online, including on the following webpages:

- www.meditateinlondon.org.uk/uk-buddhist-meditation-centres.php
- www.lbc.org.uk
- www.goingonretreat.com

- www.chezpaul.org.uk/buddhism/uk/
- www.lamrim.org.uk
- www.metta.org.uk/retreats.asp
- www.guardian.co.uk/lifeandstyle/2011/jan/22/meditation-centres-uk

These centres are affiliated to a diverse range of spiritual traditions and movements; while these are often Buddhist, it is increasingly common to find meditative practices being offered in the context of other traditions, and indeed in a secular context. Thus, for people affiliated to other religious traditions, or indeed for people uncomfortable with religion generally, there is no need to necessarily associate meditation with Buddhism; one can meditate in whatever context one feels comfortable. For example, people who identify as Christians can practise meditation within the context of their faith, for instance through the Christian meditation movement (see www.christianmeditation.org.uk for information). For people who do not identify as religious, and who might prefer to practise in a secular context, mindfulness courses tend to be offered in a way that would appeal to such sensibilities. There are many such courses to be found in the UK (e.g., see www.bemindful.co.uk for information).

Finally, men may be encouraged and helped to create their own CoP, either in addition to or as an alternative to engaging with established centres and courses. This could be nothing more than finding one other friend with an interest in meditation, and arranging to practise together once a month, creating a community of two. Even if that was the limit of one's communal participation, it would nevertheless be very valuable. In Buddhism there is the concept of a *kalyana mitrata*, meaning 'spiritual friend' (Sangharakshita, 1993). This simply recognises the value of a friendship where each takes a mutual interest in the other's practice, development, and wellbeing generally. As we have seen, meditation can be a hard endeavour sometimes, and motivation can wane. So, a commitment to meet regularly with one or more friends can help considerably in maintaining a practice. Moreover, such CoP can function as safe spaces, away from traditional hegemonic norms, where men can feel free to develop new ways of being. In this way, little by little, men may hopefully be able to find the time, space, encouragement and support to lead happier, healthier and more fulfilling lives.

References

Abeydeera, A. (2000). The travels of Marco Polo in the land of Buddhism. In V. Elisseeff (Ed.), *The Silk Road: Highways of Culture and Commerce* (pp. 69–80). Paris: UNESCO.

Abramson, L. Y., Seligman, M. E., & Teasdale, J. D. (1978). Learned helplessness in humans: Critique and reformulation. *Journal of Abnormal Psychology, 87*(1), 49–74.

Addis, M. E. (2008). Gender and depression in men. *Clinical Psychology: Science and Practice, 15*(3), 153–168.

Addis, M. E., & Mahalik, J. R. (2003). Men, masculinity, and the contexts of help seeking. *American Psychologist, 58*(1), 5–14.

Adler, A. (1927 [1992]). *Understanding Human Nature* (C. Brett, Trans.). Oxford: Oneworld.

Adler, R. H. (2009). Engel's biopsychosocial model is still relevant today. *Journal of Psychosomatic Research, 67*(6), 607–611.

Adorno, T. W. (1973). *The Jargon of Authenticity*. London: Routledge & Kegan Paul.

Ainsworth, M. D. S., Blehar, M. C., Waters, E., & Wall, S. (1979). *Patterns of Attachment: A Psychological Study of the Strange Situation*. Hillsdale, NJ: Lawrence Erlbaum Associates.

Aldao, A., Nolen-Hoeksema, S., & Schweizer, S. (2010). Emotion-regulation strategies across psychopathology: A meta-analytic review. *Clinical Psychology Review, 30*(2), 217–237.

Alexander, C. N., Rainforth, M. V., & Gelderloos, P. (1991). Transcendental meditation, self-actualization, and psychological health: A conceptual overview and statistical meta-analysis. *Journal of Social Behavior & Personality, 6*(5), 189–248.

Allen, D. J., & Oleson, T. (1999). Shame and internalized homophobia in gay men. *Journal of Homosexuality, 37*(3), 33–43.

Allen, L. (2007). 'Sensitive and real macho all at the same time': Young heterosexual men and romance. *Men and Masculinities, 10*(2), 137–152.

American Psychiatric Association [APA] (2013). *Diagnostic and Statistical Manual of Mental Disorders* (5th ed.). Washington, DC: American Psychiatric Association.

Anderson, E. D. (2009). The maintenance of masculinity among the stakeholders of sport. *Sport Management Review, 12*(1), 3–14.

Apicella, C. L., Dreber, A., Campbell, B., Gray, P. B., Hoffman, M., & Little, A. C. (2008). Testosterone and financial risk preferences. *Evolution and Human Behavior, 29*(6), 384–390.

Appelhans, B. M., Whited, M. C., Schneider, K. L., Oleski, J., & Pagoto, S. L. (2011). Response style and vulnerability to anger-induced eating in obese adults. *Eating Behaviors, 12*(1), 9–14.

Archive of Adverts and Commercials (2002). Ford Adverts and Commercials Archive: Meditation. Retrieved 16 February 2013, from www.advertolog.com/ ford/adverts/meditation-3967305/

Archive of Adverts and Commercials (2007). Pedigree Adverts and Commercials Archive: Meditating Dog. Retrieved 16 February 2013, from www.advertolog.com/pedigree/print-outdoor/meditating-dog-11004205/

Archive of Adverts and Commercials [AAC] (2008). IKEA Adverts and Commercials Archive. Retrieved 16 February 2013, from www.advertolog.com/ikea-356105/adverts/meditation-12420655/

Archive of Adverts and Commercials (2012). XXXX: Advertising and Commercial Archives. Retrieved 16 February 2013, from www.advertolog.com/xxxx-6335855/print-outdoor/meditation-camp-16031855/

Arrindell, W. A., & Luteijn, F. (2000). Similarity between intimate partners for personality traits as related to individual levels of satisfaction with life. *Personality and Individual Differences, 28*(4), 629–637.

Ashkanasy, N. M., & Daus, C. S. (2002). Emotion in the workplace: The new challenge for managers. *The Academy of Management Executive, 16*(1), 76–86.

Ashwin, S., & Lytkina, T. (2004). Men in crisis in Russia: The role of domestic marginalization. *Gender & Society, 18*(2), 189–206.

Austin, J. H. (1998). *Zen and the Brain: Toward an Understanding of Meditation and Consciousness.* Cambridge, MA: MIT Press.

Baer, R. A. (2003). Mindfulness training as a clinical intervention: A conceptual and empirical review. *Clinical Psychology: Science and Practice, 10*(2), 125–143.

Bakan, D. (1966). *The Duality of Human Existence.* Chicago: Rand McNally.

Baron-Cohen, S., & Wheelwright, S. (2004). The empathy quotient: An investigation of adults with Asperger syndrome or high functioning autism, and normal sex differences. *Journal of Autism and Developmental Disorders, 34*(2), 163–175.

Barrett, A. E., & White, H. R. (2002). Trajectories of gender role orientations in adolescence and early adulthood: A prospective study of the mental health effects of masculinity and femininity. *Journal of Health and Social Behavior, 43*(4), 451–468.

Barrett, F. J. (1996). The organizational construction of hegemonic masculinity: The case of the US navy. *Gender, Work & Organization, 3*(3), 129–142.

Barrett, L. F., & Lindquist, K. A. (2008). The embodiment of emotion. In G. Semin & E. Smith (Eds), *Embodied Grounding: Social, Cognitive, Affective, and Neuroscience Approaches* (pp. 237–262). New York: Cambridge University Press.

Baumann, M., & Prebish, C. S. (2000). *Westward Dharma: Buddhism Beyond Asia.* London: University of California Press.

BBC (2009). Beefeaters Fired in Bullying Probe. Retrieved 19 December 2011, from http://news.bbc.co.uk/1/hi/england/london/8379326.stm

Bebbington, P. E., Dunn, G., Jenkins, R., Lewis, G., Brugha, T., Farrell, M., & Meltzer, H. (1998). The influence of age and sex on the prevalence of depressive conditions: Report from the National Survey of Psychiatric Morbidity. *Psychological Medicine, 28*(1), 9–19.

Beck, A. T., Rush, A. J., Shaw, B. F., & Emery, G. (1979). *Cognitive Therapy of Depression.* New York: Guilford.

Bell, D. N., & Blanchflower, D. G. (2010). *Recession and Unemployment in the OECD.* Paper presented at the CESifo Forum.

Bem, S. L. (1974). The measurement of psychological androgyny. *Journal of Consulting and Clinical Psychology, 42*(2), 155–162.

Benson, H., Rosner, B. A., Marzetta, B. R., & Klemchuk, H. P. (1974). Decreased blood pressure in borderline hypertensive subjects who practiced meditation. *Journal of Chronic Diseases, 27*(3), 163–169.

Benson, P. R. (2010). Coping, distress, and well-being in mothers of children with autism. *Research in Autism Spectrum Disorders, 4*(2), 217–228.

Bentham, J. (1776). *A Fragment on Government.* London.

Bernardes, S. F., & Lima, M. L. (2010). Being less of a man or less of a woman: Perceptions of chronic pain patients' gender identities. *European Journal of Pain, 14*(2), 194–199.

Billig, M. (1997). The dialogic unconscious: Psychoanalysis, discursive psychology and the nature of repression. *British Journal of Social Psychology, 36*(2), 139–159.

Biswas-Diener, R., & Diener, E. (1991). Making the best of a bad situation: Satisfaction in the slums of Calcutta. In E. Diener (Ed.), *Culture and Well-Being.* Netherlands: Springer.

Blanchflower, D. G., & Oswald, A. J. (2004). Well-being over time in Britain and the USA. *Journal of Public Economics, 88*(7–8), 1359–1386.

Blechman, E. A., & Culhane, S. E. (1993). Aggressive, depressive, and prosocial coping with affective challenges in early adolescence. *The Journal of Early Adolescence, 13*(4), 361–382.

Block, N. (1995). On a confusion about a function of consciousness. *Behavioral and Brain Sciences, 18*(2), 227–287.

Bluck, R. (2006). *British Buddhism: Teachings, Practice and Development.* Oxford: Routledge.

Bohan, J. (1996). *The Psychology of Sexual Orientation: Coming to Terms.* New York: Routledge.

Boniwell, I., Osin, E., Alex Linley, P., & Ivanchenko, G. V. (2010). A question of balance: Time perspective and well-being in British and Russian samples. *The Journal of Positive Psychology, 5*(1), 24–40.

Book, A. S., Starzyk, K. B., & Quinsey, V. L. (2001). The relationship between testosterone and aggression: A meta-analysis. *Aggression and Violent Behavior, 6*(6), 579–599.

Borgonovi, F. (2008). Doing well by doing good: The relationship between formal volunteering and self-reported health and happiness. *Social Science & Medicine, 66*(11), 2321–2334.

Borton, J. L. S., Markowitz, L. J., & Dieterich, J. (2005). Effects of suppressing negative self-referent thoughts on mood and self-esteem. *Journal of Social and Clinical Psychology, 24*(2), 172–190.

Bourdieu, P. (1986). The forms of capital. In J. G. Richardson (Ed.), *Handbook of Theory and Research for the Sociology of Education* (pp. 241–258). New York: Greenwood.

Bowen, S., Witkiewitz, K., Dillworth, T. M., Chawla, N., Simpson, T. L., Ostafin, B. D., et al. (2006). Mindfulness meditation and substance use in an incarcerated population. *Psychology of Addictive Behaviors, 20*(3), 343–347.

Bowlby, J. (1973). *Attachment and Loss: Attachment,* vol. 1. New York: Basic Books.

Brandth, B., & Haugen, M. S. (2005). Doing rural masculinity: From logging to outfield tourism. *Journal of Gender Studies, 14*(1), 13–22.

Brannon, R. (1976). The male sex role: Our culture's blueprint of manhood and what it's done for us lately. In D. S. David & R. Brannon (Eds), *The Forty-Nine Percent Majority* (pp. 14–15). Reading, MA: Addison-Wesley.

Breitbart, W., Rosenfeld, B., & Perrin, H. (2000). Depression, hopelessness, and desire for hastened death in terminally ill patients with cancer. *JAMA, 284*(22), 2907–2911.

Breuer, J., & Freud, S. (1895). *Studies on Hysteria*. Standard Edition, vol. II. London: Hogarth Press.

Breuer, J., & Freud, S. (1955). Studies on hysteria. In J. Strachey (Ed. & Trans.), *Standard Edition of the Complete Psychological Works of Sigmund Freud*, vol. 2 (pp. 1–305). London: Hogarth Press. (Original work published 1893–1895.)

Brickell, C. (2005). Masculinities, performativity, and subversion: A sociological reappraisal. *Men and Masculinities, 8*(1), 24–43.

Brickell, C. (2006). The sociological construction of gender and sexuality. *The Sociological Review, 54*(1), 87–113.

Brickman, P., & Campbell, D. T. (1971). Hedonic relativism and planning the good society. In M. Appley (Ed.), *Adaptation-Level Theory* (pp. 287–305). New York: Academic Press.

Brickman, P., Coates, D., & Janoff-Bulman, R. (1978). Lottery winners and accident victims: Is happiness relative? *Journal of Personality and Social Psychology, 36*(8), 917–927.

Broderick, P. C., & Metz, S. (2009). Learning to BREATHE: A pilot trial of a mindfulness curriculum for adolescents. *Advances in School Mental Health, 2*, 35–46.

Brown, K. W., Ryan, R. M., & Creswell, J. D. (2007). Mindfulness: Theoretical foundations and evidence for its salutary effects. *Psychological Inquiry, 18*(4), 211–237.

Brownhill, S., Wilhelm, K., Barclay, L., & Schmied, V. (2005). 'Big build': Hidden depression in men. *Australian and New Zealand Journal of Psychiatry, 39*(10), 921–931.

Bruce, A., & Davies, B. (2005). Mindfulness in hospice care: Practising meditation-in-action. *Qualitative Health Research, 15*(10), 1329–1344.

Buber, M. (1958). *I and Thou*. New York: Scrivener.

Buddha, S. (1894). *Sutra on the Contemplation of Buddha Amitayus* (J. Takakusu, Trans). Sacred Books of the East Series, vol. XLIX. Oxford: Public Domain.

Buddhanet (2013). Buddhanet: Buddha, Dharma, Education Association. Retrieved 17 February 2013, from www.buddhanet.net

The Buddhist Centre (2013). Structure: Order Members. Retrieved 17 February 2013, from http://thebuddhistcentre.com/text/order-members

Burr, V. (1995). *An Introduction to Social Construction*. New York: Routledge.

Burston, D., & Frie, R. (2006). *Psychotherapy as a Human Science*. Pittsburgh, PA: Duquesne University Press.

Butler, J. (1990). *Gender Trouble: Feminism and the Subversion of Identity*. New York: Routledge Kegan Paul.

Butler, J. (1993). *Bodies that Matter: On the Discursive Limits of 'Sex'*. New York: Routledge.

Cahn, B. R., & Polich, J. (2006). Meditation states and traits: EEG, ERP, and neuroimaging studies. *Psychological Bulletin, 132*(2), 180–211.

Campbell, A. (2008). Attachment, aggression and affiliation: The role of oxytocin in female social behavior. *Biological Psychology, 77*(1), 1–10.

Campbell, C. (2004). I shop therefore I know that I am: The metaphysical basis of modern consumerism. In K. M. Ekström & H. Brembeck (Eds), *Elusive Consumption* (pp. 27–43). Oxford: Berg.

Campbell, C. A. (1995). Male gender roles and sexuality: Implications for women's AIDS risk and prevention. *Social Science & Medicine, 41*(2), 197–210.

Camus, A. (1942). *The Stranger* (S. Gilbert, Trans.). New York: Vintage Books.

Cardoso, R., de Souza, E., Camano, L., & Roberto Leite, J. (2004). Meditation in health: An operational definition. *Brain Research Protocols, 14*(1), 58–60.

Carlisle, S., Henderson, G., & Hanlon, P. W. (2009). 'Wellbeing': A collateral casualty of modernity? *Social Science & Medicine, 69*(10), 1556–1560.

Carver, C. S., & Scheier, M. F. (1998). *On the Self Regulation of Behavior*. Cambridge: Cambridge University Press.

Carver, C. S., Scheier, M. F., & Weintraub, J. K. (1989). Assessing coping strategies: A theoretically based approach. *Journal of Personality and Social Psychology, 56*(2), 267–283.

Chancellor, J., & Lyubomirsky, S. (2011). Happiness and thrift: When (spending) less is (hedonically) more. *Journal of Consumer Psychology, 21*(2), 131–138.

Chaplin, T. M., Cole, P. M., & Zahn-Waxler, C. (2005). Parental socialization of emotion expression: Gender differences and relations to child adjustment. *Emotion, 5*(1), 80–88.

Chapman, A. L., Specht, M. W., & Cellucci, T. (2005). Borderline personality disorder and deliberate self-harm: Does experiential avoidance play a role? *Suicide and Life-Threatening Behavior, 35*(4), 388–399.

Chiesa, A., Calati, R., & Serretti, A. (2011). Does mindfulness training improve cognitive abilities? A systematic review of neuropsychological findings. *Clinical Psychology Review, 31*(3), 449–464.

Chryssides, G. D., & Wilkins, M. Z. (2006). *A Reader in New Religious Movements*. London: Continuum.

Chwalisz, K., Diener, E., & Gallagher, D. (1988). Autonomic arousal feedback and emotional experience: Evidence from the spinal cord injured. *Journal of Personality and Social Psychology, 54*(5), 820–828.

Clark, A., Knabe, A., & Rätzel, S. (2010). Boon or bane? Others' unemployment, well-being and job insecurity. *Labour Economics, 17*(1), 52–61.

CNN (2012). Fighting Loneliness and Disease with Meditation. 25 August 2012, retrieved 16 February 2013, from http://edition.cnn.com/2012/08/25/health/meditation-loneliness-inflammation-enayati

Cochran, S. V., & Rabinowitz, F. E. (2000). *Men and Depression: Clinical and Empirical Perspectives*. San Diego: Academic Press.

Cohen, E. (2010). From the Bodhi tree to the analyst's couch, then into the MRI scanner: The psychologisation of Buddhism. *Annual Review of Critical Psychology, 8*, 97–119.

Cohen, S. A. (2011). Lifestyle travellers: Backpacking as a way of life. *Annals of Tourism Research, 38*(4), 1535–1555.

Connell, R. W. (1995). *Masculinities*. Berkeley: University of California Press.

Connell, R. W., & Messerschmidt, J. W. (2005). Hegemonic masculinity: Rethinking the concept. *Gender & Society, 19*(6), 829–859.

Connell, R. W., & Wood, J. (2005). Globalization and business masculinities. *Men and Masculinities, 7*(4), 347–364.

Cooper, C. L., & Cartwright, S. (1994). Healthy mind, healthy organization: A proactive approach to occupational stress. *Human Relations, 47*(4), 455–471.

Coren, S. (1998). Prenatal testosterone exposure, left-handedness, and high school delinquency. *Behavioral and Brain Sciences, 21*(03), 369–370.

Courtenay, W. H. (1998). College men's health: An overview and a call to action. *Journal of American College Health, 46*(6), 279–290.

Courtenay, W. H. (2000). Constructions of masculinity and their influence on men's well-being: A theory of gender and health. *Social Science & Medicine, 50*(10), 1385–1401.

Cousins, L. S. (1996). The dating of the historical Buddha: A review article. *Journal of the Royal Asiatic Society (Third Series), 6*(1), 57–63.

Covert, B. (2012). Memo to Corporate America: More Women Leaders Means a Better Bottom Line. *Forbes*, 1 August.

Coyle, A. (2008). Qualitative methods and 'the (partly) ineffable' in psychological research on religion and spirituality. *Qualitative Research in Psychology, 5*(1), 56–67.

Cramer, K. M., Gallant, M. D., & Langlois, M. W. (2005). Self-silencing and depression in women and men: Comparative structural equation models. *Personality and Individual Differences, 39*(3), 581–592.

Creighton, G. (2011). *Troubled masculinity: Exploring gender identity and risk-taking following the death of a friend.* (PhD), University of British Columbia, Electronic Theses and Dissertations. Retrieved from https://circle.ubc.ca/handle/2429/37961

Crowther-Heyck, H. (1999). George A. Miller, language, and the computer metaphor and mind. *History of Psychology, 2*(1), 37–64.

Csikszentmihalyi, M. (1990). *Flow: The Psychology of Optimal Experience.* New York: Harper Perennial.

Curley, A. J. (2012). Gender Testing 'Imperfect' for Female Athletes. *Expert*, 8 August 2012, retrieved 10 January 2013, from cnn.co.uk

Cutcliffe, J. R. (2005). Adapt or adopt: Developing and transgressing the methodological boundaries of grounded theory. *Journal of Advanced Nursing, 51*(4), 421–428.

Danna, K., & Griffin, R. W. (1999). Health and well-being in the workplace: A review and synthesis of the literature. *Journal of Management, 25*(3), 357–384.

D'Augelli, A. R., Grossman, A. H., Hershberger, S. L., & O'Connell, T. S. (2001). Aspects of mental health among older lesbian, gay, and bisexual adults. *Aging & Mental Health, 5*(2), 149–158.

Davidson, K. (2004). 'Why can't a man be more like a woman?': Marital status and social networking of older men. *The Journal of Men's Studies, 13*(1), 25–43.

Dawson, L. L. (1998). Anti-modernism, modernism, and postmodernism: Struggling with the cultural significance of new religious movements. *Sociology of Religion, 59*(2), 131–156.

Day, A. L., & Carroll, S. A. (2004). Using an ability-based measure of emotional intelligence to predict individual performance, group performance, and group citizenship behaviours. *Personality and Individual Differences, 36*(6), 1443–1458.

de Chavez, A. C., Backett-Milburn, K., Parry, O., & Platt, S. (2005). Understanding and researching wellbeing: Its usage in different disciplines and potential for health research and health promotion. *Health Education Journal, 64*(1), 70–87.

de Pillis, E., & de Pillis, L. (2008). Are engineering schools masculine and authoritarian? The mission statements say yes. *Journal of Diversity in Higher Education, 1*(1), 33.

de Saussure, F. (1916). *Course in General Linguistics.* New York: Philosophical Library.

de Visser, R. O., & Smith, J. A. (2007). Alcohol consumption and masculine identity among young men. *Psychology & Health, 22*(5), 595–614.

de Visser, R. O., Smith, J. A., & McDonnell, E. J. (2009). 'That's not masculine': Masculine capital and health-related behaviour. *Journal of Health Psychology, 14*(7), 1047–1058.

Dennett, D. (1990). *Consciousness Explained.* London: Allen Lane.

Denzin, N. K. (1985). Emotion as lived experience. *Symbolic Interaction, 8*(2), 223–240.

Derrida, J. (1982). *Margins of Philosophy.* Chicago: University of Chicago Press.

Descartes, R. (1641 [2008]). *Meditations on First Philosophy: With Selections from the Objections and Replies* (M. Moriarty, Trans.). Oxford: Oxford University Press.

Diener, E., & Emmons, R. A. (1984). The independence of positive and negative affect. *Journal of Personality and Social Psychology, 47*(5), 1105–1117.

Diener, E., & Oishi, S. (2000). Money and happiness: Income and subjective well-being across nations. In E. Diener & E. M. Suh (Eds), *Culture and Subjective Well-Being* (pp. 185–218). Cambridge, MA: MIT Press.

Diener, E., Suh, E. M., Lucas, R. E., & Smith, H. L. (1999). Subjective well-being: Three decades of progress. *Psychological Bulletin, 125*(2), 276–302.

Diener, E., Gohm, C. L., Suh, E., & Oishi, S. (2000). Similarity of the relations between marital status and subjective well-being across cultures. *Journal of Cross-Cultural Psychology, 31*(4), 419–436.

Digeser, P. (1994). Performativity trouble: Postmodern feminism and essential subjects. *Political Research Quarterly, 47*(3), 655–673.

Dillard-Wright, D. B., & Jerath, D. (2011). *The Everything Guide to Meditation for Healthy Living.* Avon, MA: Adams Media.

Dimitriadis, G. (2009). *Performing Identity/Performing Culture: Hip Hop as Text, Pedagogy, and Lived Practice.* New York: Peter Lang Publishing.

Ditto, B., Eclache, M., & Goldman, N. (2006). Short-term autonomic and cardiovascular effects of mindfulness body scan meditation. *Annals of Behavioral Medicine, 32*(3), 227–234.

Dobkin, P. L., Irving, J. A., & Amar, S. (2012). For whom may participation in a mindfulness-based stress reduction program be contraindicated? *Mindfulness, 3*(1), 44–50.

Doyle, L., & Gough, I. (1991). *A Theory of Human Need.* London: Macmillan.

Duff, P. A., & Bell, J. S. (2002). Narrative research in TESOL: Narrative inquiry: More than just telling stories. *TESOL Quarterly, 36*(2), 207–213.

Dumoulin, H. (1979). *Zen Enlightenment: Origins and Meaning.* New York: Wetherhill.

Eagly, A. H., & Wood, W. (1999). The origins of sex differences in human behavior: Evolved dispositions versus social roles. *American Psychologist, 54*(6), 408–423.

Easterlin, R. A. (1995). Will raising the incomes of all increase the happiness of all? *Journal of Economic Behavior & Organization, 27*(1), 35–47.

Eckert, P., & McConnell-Ginet, S. (1992). Think practically and look locally: Language and gender as community-based practice. *Annual Review of Anthropology, 21*, 461–490.

Economic and Human Rights Commission [EHRC] (2011). How Fair is Britain? Equality, Human Rights and Good Relations in 2010. *Triennial Review 2010.*

Edwards, D. A., Wetzel, K., & Wyner, D. R. (2006). Intercollegiate soccer: Saliva cortisol and testosterone are elevated during competition, and testosterone is related to status and social connectedness with teammates. *Physiology & Behavior, 87*(1), 135–143.

Eichstedt, J. A., Serbin, L. A., Poulin-Dubois, D., & Sen, M. G. (2002). Of bears and men: Infants' knowledge of conventional and metaphorical gender stereotypes. *Infant Behavior and Development, 25*(3), 296–310.

Engel, G. L. (1977). The need for a new medical model: A challenge for biomedicine. *Science, 196*(4286), 129–136.

Epstein, M. (1988). The deconstruction of the self: Ego and 'egolessness' in Buddhist insight meditation. *The Journal of Transpersonal Psychology, 20*(1), 61–69.

Erricker, C., & Erricker, J. (2001). *Meditation in Schools: A Practical Guide to Calmer Classrooms*. New York: Continuum.

Farrell, M., Howes, S., Bebbington, P., Brugha, T., Jenkins, R., Lewis, G., et al. (2001). Nicotine, alcohol and drug dependence and psychiatric comorbidity: Results of a national household survey. *British Journal of Psychiatry, 179*, 432–437.

Faure, B. (2003). *The Power of Denial: Buddhism, Purity, and Gender*. Princeton: Princeton University Press.

Fell, J. (2004). Identifying neural correlates of consciousness: The state space approach. *Consciousness and Cognition, 13*(4), 709–729.

Ferrer-i-Carbonell, A. (2005). Income and well-being: An empirical analysis of the comparison income effect. *Journal of Public Economics, 89*(5–6), 997–1019.

Fine, C. (2008). Will working mothers' brains explode? The popular new genre of neurosexism. *Neuroethics, 1*(1), 69–72.

Finlay, B., & Walther, C. S. (2003). The relation of religious affiliation, service attendance, and other factors to homophobic attitudes among university students. *Review of Religious Research*, 370–393.

Fisher, R. (2006). Still thinking: The case for meditation with children. *Thinking Skills and Creativity, 1*(2), 146–151.

Flood, M. (2003). Lust, trust and latex: Why young heterosexual men do not use condoms. *Culture, Health & Sexuality, 5*(4), 353–369.

Fowler, R. D., Seligman, M. E. P., & Koocher, G. P. (1999). The APA 1998 Annual Report. *American Psychologist, 54*(8), 537–568.

Francis, B. (1999). Lads, lasses and (New) Labour: 14–16-year-old students' responses to the 'laddish behaviour and boys' underachievement' debate. *British Journal of Sociology of Education, 20*(3), 355–371.

Frank, W. S. (1997). *The Wounded Storyteller: Body, Illness and Ethics*. Chicago: University of Chicago Press.

Fredrickson, B. L. (2001). The role of positive emotions in positive psychology: The broaden-and-build theory of positive emotions. *American Psychologist, 56*(3), 218–226.

Fredrickson, B. L., Cohn, M. A., Coffey, K. A., Pek, J., & Finkel, S. M. (2008). Open hearts build lives: Positive emotions, induced through loving-kindness meditation, build consequential personal resources. *Journal of Personality and Social Psychology, 95*(5), 1045–1062.

Fresco, D. M., Moore, M. T., van Dulmen, M. H. M., Segal, Z. V., Ma, S. H., Teasdale, J. D., & Williams, J. M. G. (2007). Initial psychometric properties of the experiences questionnaire: Validation of a self-report measure of decentering. *Behavior Therapy, 38*(3), 234–246.

Freud, S. (1914). *On the History of the Psychoanalytic Movement.* Standard Edition, vol. XIV. London: Hogarth Press.

Freud, S. (1915). *Repression.* Standard Edition, vol. XIV. London: Hogarth Press.

Freud, S. (1918). *From the History of an Infantile Neurosis.* Standard Edition, vol. III. London: Hogarth Press.

Freud, S. (1949). *The Ego and the Id.* Standard Edition, vol. XIX. London: Hogarth Press.

Frosh, S., Phoenix, A., & Pattman, R. (2003). The trouble with boys. *The Psychologist, 16*(2), 84–87.

Frost, N., Nolas, S. M., Brooks-Gordon, B., Esin, C., Holt, A., Mehdizadeh, L., & Shinebourne, P. (2010). Pluralism in qualitative research: The impact of different researchers and qualitative approaches on the analysis of qualitative data. *Qualitative Research, 10*(4), 1–20.

Galdas, P. M., Cheater, F., & Marshall, P. (2005). Men and health help-seeking behaviour: Literature review. *Journal of Advanced Nursing, 49*(6), 616–623.

Gallagher, S. (2000). Philosophical conceptions of the self: Implications for cognitive science. *Trends in Cognitive Sciences, 4*(1), 14–21.

Ganster, D. C., & Victor, B. (1988). The impact of social support on mental and physical health. *British Journal of Medical Psychology, 61*(1), 17–36.

Geary, D. C. (1998). *Male, Female: The Evolution of Human Sex Differences.* Washington, DC: American Psychological Association.

George, J. M., & Jones, G. R. (1996). The experience of work and turnover intentions: Interactive effects of value attainment, job satisfaction, and positive mood. *Journal of Applied Psychology, 81*(3), 318–325.

Gergen, K. (2001). The dissolution of the self. In E. Ksenych & D. Liu (Eds), *Conflict, Order and Action: Readings in Sociology* (3rd ed., pp. 431–441). Toronto, Ontario: Canadian Scholars' Press.

Gerson, J. M., & Peiss, K. (1985). Boundaries, negotiation, consciousness: Reconceptualizing gender relations. *Social Problems, 32*(4), 317–331.

Giddens, A., & Dallmayr, F. R. (1982). *Profiles and Critiques in Social Theory.* Berkeley: University of California Press.

Gilbert, P. (2005). *Compassion: Conceptualisations, Research and Use in Psychotherapy.* Hove, East Sussex: Routledge.

Gilmartin, S. K. (2007). Crafting heterosexual masculine identities on campus: College men talk about romantic love. *Men and Masculinities, 9*(4), 530–539.

Glaser, B. G., & Strauss, A. L. (1967). *The Discovery of Grounded Theory: Strategies for Qualitative Research.* Chicago: Aldine.

Goldberg, D., & Huxley, P. (1992). *Common Mental Disorders: A Bio-social Model.* London: Tavistock.

Golding, B., Kimberley, H., Foley, A., & Brown, M. (2008). Houses and sheds in Australia: An exploration of the genesis and growth of neighbourhood houses and men's sheds in community settings. *Australian Journal of Adult Learning, 48*(2), 237–262.

Goleman, D. (1988). *The Meditative Mind: The Varieties of Meditative Experience.* New York: Tarcher.

Goleman, D. (1995). *Emotional Intelligence: Why it can Matter more than IQ.* New York: Bantam Books.

Gonçalves, Ó. F. (1994). From epistemological truth to existential meaning in cognitive narrative psychotherapy. *Journal of Constructivist Psychology, 7*(2), 107–118.

Goodenough, U., & Woodruff, P. (2001). Mindful virtue, mindful reverence. *Zygon, 36*(4), 585–595.

Gough, B. (2001). 'Biting your tongue': Negotiating masculinities in contemporary Britain. *Journal of Gender Studies, 10*(2), 169–185.

Gough, B. (2006). Try to be healthy, but don't forgo your masculinity: Deconstructing men's health discourse in the media. *Social Science & Medicine, 63*(9), 2476–2488.

Gough, B. (2007). 'Real men don't diet': An analysis of contemporary newspaper representations of men, food and health. *Social Science & Medicine, 64*(2), 326–337.

Gramsci, A. (1971). *Selections from the Prison Notebooks.* New York: International.

Granié, M.-A. (2010). Gender stereotype conformity and age as determinants of preschoolers' injury-risk behaviors. *Accident Analysis & Prevention, 42*(2), 726–733.

Graves, C. W. (1970). Levels of existence: An open system theory of values. *Journal of Humanistic Psychology, 10*(2), 131–155.

Green, D. P., & Salovey, P. (1999). In what sense are positive and negative affect independent? A reply to Tellegen, Watson, and Clark. *Psychological Science, 10*(4), 304–306.

Green, G., Emslie, C., O'Neill, D., Hunt, K., & Walker, S. (2010). Exploring the ambiguities of masculinity in accounts of emotional distress in the military among young ex-servicemen. *Social Science & Medicine, 71*(8), 1480–1488.

Greenberg, L. S. (2004). Emotion-focused therapy. *Clinical Psychology & Psychotherapy, 11*(1), 3–16.

Gross, J. J. (1999). Emotion regulation: Past, present, future. *Cognition & Emotion, 13*(5), 551–573.

The Guardian (2013). Life & Style: Meditation. Retrieved 16 February 2013, from www.guardian.co.uk/lifeandstyle/meditation

Guasp, A. (2012). *The School Report: The Experiences of Gay Young People in Britain's Schools in 2012.* Cambridge: Stonewall.

Gyatso, G. K. (2007). *Introduction to Buddhism: An Explanation of the Buddhist Way of Life.* New York: Tharpa Publications.

Gyatso, G. K. (2009). *Eight Steps to Happiness: The Buddhist Way of Loving Kindness.* New York: Tharpa Publications.

Gyatso, T. (2006). Science at the crossroads. *Explore: The Journal of Science and Healing, 2*(2), 97–99.

Hagerty, M. R. (2000). Social comparisons of income in one's community: Evidence from national surveys of income and happiness. *Journal of Personality and Social Psychology, 78*(4), 764–771.

Hankivsky, O., & Christoffersen, A. (2008). Intersectionality and the determinants of health: A Canadian perspective. *Critical Public Health, 18*(3), 271–283.

Harris, A. P. (2000). Gender, violence, race, and criminal justice. *Stanford Law Review, 52*(4), 777–807.

Harrison, P. A. (2004). *Elements of Pantheism: Religious Reverence of Nature and the Universe.* New York: Llumina Press.

Hart, W. (1987). *The Art of Living: Vipassana Meditation as Taught by Goenka.* New York: HarperOne.

Harvey, P. (1990). *An Introduction to Buddhism: Teachings, History and Practices.* Cambridge: Cambridge University Press.

Harvey, S. (1999). Hegemonic masculinity, friendship, and group formation in an athletic subculture. *The Journal of Men's Studies, 8*(1), 91–108.

Hasanović, M., Sinanović, O., Pajević, I., & Agius, M. (2011). The spiritual approach to group psychotherapy treatment of psychotraumatized persons in post-war Bosnia and Herzegovina. *Religions, 2*(3), 330–344.

Hassmén, P., Koivula, N., & Uutela, A. (2000). Physical exercise and psychological well-being: A population study in Finland. *Preventive Medicine, 30*(1), 17–25.

Hatch, S. L., Harvey, S. B., & Maughan, B. (2010). A developmental-contextual approach to understanding mental health and well-being in early adulthood. *Social Science & Medicine, 70*(2), 261–268.

Hay, I., Ashman, A. F., & Van Kraayenoord, C. E. (1998). The influence of gender, academic achievement and non-school factors upon pre-adolescent self-concept. *Educational Psychology, 18*(4), 461–470.

Hayes, R. (1995). Androgyny Among Friends. Retrieved from www.unm.edu/~ rhayes/afterpat.pd

Hayes, S. C. (2002). Buddhism and acceptance and commitment therapy. *Cognitive and Behavioral Practice, 9*(1), 58–66.

Headey, B., Schupp, J., Tucci, I., & Wagner, G. G. (2010). Authentic happiness theory supported by impact of religion on life satisfaction: A longitudinal analysis with data for Germany. *The Journal of Positive Psychology, 5*(1), 73–82.

Hearn, J. (1997). The implications of critical studies on men. *NORA – Nordic Journal of Feminist and Gender Research, 5*(1), 48–60.

Heidegger, M. (1927). *Being and Time* (J. MacQuarrie & E. Robinson, Trans.). London: Blackwell.

Helliwell, J. F., & Putnam, R. D. (2004). The social context of well-being. *Philosophical Transactions of the Royal Society of London. Series B: Biological Sciences, 359*(1449), 1435–1446.

Hilti, C. C., Hilti, L. M., Heinemann, D., Robbins, T., Seifritz, E., & Cattapan-Ludewig, K. (2010). Impaired performance on the Rapid Visual Information Processing task (RVIP) could be an endophenotype of schizophrenia. *Psychiatry Research, 177*(1–2), 60–64.

Hochschild, A. R. (1979). Emotion work, feeling rules, and social structure. *American Journal of Sociology, 85*(3), 551–575.

Holmes, T. H., & Rahe, R. H. (1967). The social readjustment rating scale. *Journal of Psychosomatic Research, 11*(2), 213–218.

Honkalampi, K., Hintikka, J., Tanskanen, A., Lehtonen, J., & Viinamäki, H. (2000). Depression is strongly associated with alexithymia in the general population. *Journal of Psychosomatic Research, 48*(1), 99–104.

Horton, S. (2008). Consuming childhood: 'Lost' and 'ideal' childhoods as a motivation for migration. *Anthropological Quarterly, 81*(4), 925–943.

Hume, D. (1739). *A Treatise of Human Nature.* Oxford: Clarendon Press.

Huta, V., & Ryan, R. (2010). Pursuing pleasure or virtue: The differential and overlapping well-being benefits of hedonic and eudaimonic motives. *Journal of Happiness Studies, 11*(6), 735–762.

Irving, J. A., Dobkin, P. L., & Park, J. (2009). Cultivating mindfulness in health care professionals: A review of empirical studies of mindfulness-based stress reduction (MBSR). *Complementary Therapies in Clinical Practice, 15*(2), 61–66.

Ivakhiv, A. (2003). Orchestrating sacred space: Beyond the social construction of nature. *Ecotheology, 8*(1), 11–29.

Jackson, C. (2002). 'Laddishness' as a self-worth protection strategy. *Gender and Education, 14*(1), 37–50.

Jackson, C., & Dempster, S. (2009). 'I sat back on my computer…with a bottle of whisky next to me': Constructing 'cool' masculinity through 'effortless' achievement in secondary and higher education. *Journal of Gender Studies, 18*(4), 341–356.

Janoff-Bulman, R., & Yopyk, D. J. (2004). Random outcomes and valued commitments. In J. Greenberg, S. L. Koole, & T. Pyszczynski (Eds), *Handbook of Experimental Existential Psychology* (pp. 122–140). New York: Guilford.

Jaspers, K. (1986). *Basic Philosophical Writings* (E. Ehrlich, L. H. Ehrlich, & G. B. Pepper, Eds). Athens: Ohio University Press.

Jenning, J. (1999). Structuralism. In S. Glendinning (Ed.), *The Edinburgh Encyclopedia of Continental Philosophy* (pp. 502–514). Edinburgh: Fitzroy Dearborn Publishers.

Johnson, D. P., Penn, D. L., Fredrickson, B. L., Meyer, P. S., Kring, A. M., & Brantley, M. (2009). Loving-kindness meditation to enhance recovery from negative symptoms of schizophrenia. *Journal of Clinical Psychology, 65*(5), 499–509.

Jones, G. (2002). *The Youth Divide: Diverging Paths to Adulthood.* York: York Publishing Services for the Joseph Rowntree Foundation.

Jones, S. (2003). *Y: The Descent of Man.* Boston: Houghton Mifflin.

Jorgensen, B. S., Jamieson, R. D., & Martin, J. F. (2010). Income, sense of community and subjective well-being: Combining economic and psychological variables. *Journal of Economic Psychology, 31*(4), 612–623.

Josipovic, Z. (2010). Duality and nonduality in meditation research. *Consciousness and Cognition, 19*(4), 1119–1121.

Judiciary of England and Wales (2012). 2012 Judicial Diversity Statistics – Gender, Ethnicity, Profession and Age.

Jung, C. G. (1951). Aion. *The Collected Works of C. G. Jung,* vol. IX. London: Routledge and Kegan Paul.

Kabat-Zinn, J. (1982). An outpatient program in behavioral medicine for chronic pain patients based on the practice of mindfulness meditation: Theoretical considerations and preliminary results. *General Hospital Psychiatry, 4*(1), 33–47.

Kabat-Zinn, J. (2003). Mindfulness-based interventions in context: Past, present, and future. *Clinical Psychology: Science and Practice, 10*(2), 144–156.

Kaiseler, M., Polman, R., & Nicholls, A. (2009). Mental toughness, stress, stress appraisal, coping and coping effectiveness in sport. *Personality and Individual Differences, 47*(7), 728–733.

Kang, C. (2009). Buddhist and Tantric perspectives on causality and society. *Journal of Buddhist Ethics, 16*, 69–103.

Kaplan, A. (1989). *Meditation and Kabbalah.* Boston: Weiser Books.

Karasek, R. A. (1997). Demand/control model: A social, emotional, and physiological approach to stress risk and active behavior development. In J. M. Stellman (Ed.), *ILO Encyclopedia of Occupational Health and Safety* (p. 34). Geneva: ILO.

Kenway, J., & Fitzclarence, L. (1997). Masculinity, violence and schooling: Challenging 'poisonous pedagogies'. *Gender and Education, 9*(1), 117–134.

Kessler, R. C. (2003). Epidemiology of women and depression. *Journal of Affective Disorders, 74*(1), 5–13.

Kessler, R. C., Berglund, P., Demler, O., Jin, R., Merikangas, K. R., & Walters, E. E. (2005). Lifetime prevalence and age-of-onset distributions of DSM-IV disorders in the National Comorbidity Survey Replication. *Archives of General Psychiatry, 62*(6), 593–602.

Keyes, C. L. M., Shmotkin, D., & Ryff, C. D. (2002). Optimizing well-being: The empirical encounter of two traditions. *Journal of Personality and Social Psychology, 82*(6), 1007–1022.

Kiefer, I., Rathmanner, T., & Kunze, M. (2005). Eating and dieting differences in men and women. *The Journal of Men's Health & Gender, 2*(2), 194–201.

Kierkegaard, S. (1843). *Fear and Trembling and the Sickness unto Death* (M. Lowrie, Trans.). Princeton, NJ: Princeton University Press.

Kilmartin, C. (2005). Depression in men: Communication, diagnosis and therapy. *The Journal of Men's Health & Gender, 2*(1), 95–99.

Kilminster, S., Downes, J., Gough, B., Murdoch-Eaton, D., & Roberts, T. (2007). Women in medicine – is there a problem? A literature review of the changing gender composition, structures and occupational cultures in medicine. *Medical Education, 41*(1), 39–49.

Kiselica, M. S., & Englar-Carlson, M. (2010). Identifying, affirming, and building upon male strengths: The positive psychology/positive masculinity model of psychotherapy with boys and men. *Psychotherapy: Theory, Research, Practice, Training, 47*(3), 276–287.

Kiyota, M. (1978). *Mahayana Buddhist Meditation: Theory and Practice.* Hawaii: University Press.

Koch, C., & Tsuchiya, N. (2007). Attention and consciousness: Two distinct brain processes. *Trends in Cognitive Sciences, 11*(1), 16.

Koenig, H. G. (2009). Research on religion, spirituality, and mental health: A review. *Canadian Journal of Psychiatry, 54*(5), 283–291.

Kohlberg, L. (1968). Stage and sequence: The cognitive-developmental approach to socialization. In D. A. Goslin (Ed.), *Handbook of Socialization Theory and Research* (pp. 347–480). London: Rand McNally.

Kramer, K. (1988). *The Sacred Art of Dying: How World Religions Understand Death.* Mahwah, NJ: Paulist Press.

Kristeller, J. L., & Hallett, C. B. (1999). An exploratory study of a meditation-based intervention for binge eating disorder. *Journal of Health Psychology, 4*(3), 357–363.

Kuijpersa, H. J. H., van der Heijdena, F. M. M. A., Tuiniera, S., & Verhoeven, W. M. A. (2007). Meditation-induced psychosis. *Psychopathology, 40*(6), 461–464.

Kulis, S., Marsiglia, F. F., Lingard, E. C., Nieri, T., & Nagoshi, J. (2008). Gender identity and substance use among students in two high schools in Monterrey, Mexico. *Drug and Alcohol Dependence, 95*(3), 260.

Kumar, S. M. (2002). An introduction to Buddhism for the cognitive-behavioral therapist. *Cognitive and Behavioral Practice, 9*(1), 40–43.

Labouvie, E., & Bates, M. E. (2002). Reasons for alcohol use in young adulthood: Validation of a three-dimensional measure. *Journal of Studies on Alcohol, 63*(2), 145–155.

Larson, J. S. (1999). The conceptualization of health. *Medical Care Research and Review, 56*(2), 123–136.

LaSala, M. C. (2000). Lesbians, gay men, and their parents: Family therapy for the coming-out crisis. *Family Process, 39*(1), 67–81.

Lave, J., & Wenger, E. (1991). *Situated Learning: Legitimate Peripheral Participation.* Cambridge: Cambridge University Press.

Lawler-Row, K. A. (2010). Forgiveness as a mediator of the religiosity–health relationship. *Psychology of Religion and Spirituality, 2*(1), 1–16.

Lazarus, R. S., & Folkman, S. (1987). Transactional theory and research on emotions and coping. *European Journal of Personality, 1*(3), 141–169.

Lee, W. R., McQuellon, R. P., Harris-Henderson, K., Case, L. D., & McCullough, D. L. (2000). A preliminary analysis of health-related quality of life in the first year after permanent source interstitial brachytherapy (PIB) for clinically localized prostate cancer. *International Journal of Radiation Oncology, Biology, Physics, 46*(1), 77–81.

Levant, R. F. (1992). Toward the reconstruction of masculinity. *Journal of Family Psychology, 5*(3–4), 379–402.

Levant, R. F. (1998). *Desperately Seeking Language: Understanding, Assessing, and Treating Normative Male Alexithymia.* New York: John Wiley & Sons Inc.

Levant, R. F., Hall, R. J., Williams, C. M., & Hasan, N. T. (2009). Gender differences in alexithymia. *Psychology of Men & Masculinity, 10*(3), 190–203.

Lévi-Strauss, C. (1981). *The Naked Man.* Chicago: University of Chicago Press.

Lewisohn, L. (1997). The sacred music of Islam: Samā' in the Persian Sufi tradition. *British Journal of Ethnomusicology, 6*(1), 1–33.

Lindkvist, L. (2005). Knowledge communities and knowledge collectivities: A typology of knowledge work in groups. *Journal of Management Studies, 42*(6), 1189–1210.

Linley, P. A., & Joseph, S. (2004). Applied positive psychology: A new perspective for professional practice. In P. A. Linley & S. Joseph (Eds), *Positive Psychology in Practice* (pp. 3–12). Hoboken, NJ: John Wiley and Sons.

Lock, A., & Strong, T. (2010). *Social Constructionism: Sources and Stirrings in Theory and Practice.* Cambridge: Cambridge University Press.

Lokhabandhu, D. (2007). Perspectives on Friends of the Western Buddhist Order: Some Facts and Figures. Retrieved from http://discussion.fwbo.org/western-buddhist-order/the-western-buddhist-order-some-facts-and-figures

Lomas, T. (2013). Critical positive masculinity. *Masculinities and Social Change, 2*(2), 167–193.

Lomas, T., Cartwright, T., Edginton, T., & Ridge, D. (2013). Engagement with meditation as a positive health trajectory: Divergent narratives of progress in male meditators. *Psychology and Health.* doi: 10.1080/08870446.2013.843684

Lonczak, H. S., Neighbors, C., & Donovan, D. M. (2007). Predicting risky and angry driving as a function of gender. *Accident Analysis & Prevention, 39*(3), 536–545.

Lorber, J. (1996). Beyond the binaries: Depolarising the categories of sex, sexuality and gender. *Sociological Inquiry, 66*(2), 143–160.

Lucas, R. E., & Schimmack, U. (2009). Income and well-being: How big is the gap between the rich and the poor? *Journal of Research in Personality, 43*(1), 75–78.

Lucas, R. E., Clark, A. E., Georgellis, Y., & Diener, E. (2004). Unemployment alters the set point for life satisfaction. *Psychological Science, 15*(1), 8–13.

Luginaah, I. N., Taylor, S. M., Elliott, S. J., & Eyles, J. D. (2002). Community responses and coping strategies in the vicinity of a petroleum refinery in Oakville, Ontario. *Health & Place, 8*(3), 177–190.

Lund, C., Breen, A., Flisher, A. J., Kakuma, R., Corrigall, J., Joska, J. A., et al. (2010). Poverty and common mental disorders in low and middle income countries: A systematic review. *Social Science & Medicine, 71*(3), 517–528.

Lupton, D. (1998). *The Emotional Self*. London: Sage.

Lustyk, M. K., Chawla, N., Nolan, R. S., & Marlatt, G. A. (2009). Mindfulness meditation research: Issues of participant screening, safety procedures, and researcher training. *Advances in Mind-Body Medicine, 24*(1), 20–30.

Lutz, A., Slagter, H. A., Dunne, J. D., & Davidson, R. J. (2008). Attention regulation and monitoring in meditation. *Trends in Cognitive Sciences, 12*(4), 163–169.

Lutze, F. E., & Bell, C. A. (2005). Boot camp prisons as masculine organizations. *Journal of Offender Rehabilitation, 40*(3–4), 133–152.

Lykken, D., & Tellegen, A. (1996). Happiness is a stochastic phenomenon. *Psychological Science, 7*(3), 186–189.

Lyubomirsky, S., Sheldon, K. M., & Schkade, D. (2005). Pursuing happiness: The architecture of sustainable change. *Review of General Psychology, 9*(2), 111–131.

Ma, S. H., & Teasdale, J. D. (2004). Mindfulness-based cognitive therapy for depression: Replication and exploration of differential relapse prevention effects. *Journal of Consulting and Clinical Psychology, 72*(1), 31–40.

Mac an Ghaill, M., & Haywood, C. (2012). Understanding boys: Thinking through boys, masculinity and suicide. *Social Science & Medicine, 74*(4), 482–489.

Maccoby, E. E., & Jacklin, C. N. (1974). *The Psychology of Sex Differences* (Vol. 1). Stanford, CA: Stanford University Press.

Marchand, A., Demers, A., & Durand, P. (2005). Does work really cause distress? The contribution of occupational structure and work organization to the experience of psychological distress. *Social Science & Medicine, 61*(1), 1–14.

Markus, H. R., & Herzog, A. R. (1991). The role of the self-concept in aging. *Annual Review of Gerontology and Geriatrics, 11*, 110–143.

Mars, T. S., & Abbey, H. (2010). Mindfulness meditation practise as a healthcare intervention: A systematic review. *International Journal of Osteopathic Medicine, 13*(2), 56–66.

Marshall, J. D. (2010). Introduction. In J. D. Marshall (Ed.), *Poststructuralism, Philosophy, Pedagogy* (pp. xiii–xxvi). Netherlands: Kluwer Academic Publishers.

Maslow, A. H. (1943). A theory of human motivation. *Psychological Review, 50*(4), 370–396.

Masten, J. (1994). My two dads: Collaboration and the reproduction of Beaumont and Fletcher. In J. Goldberg (Ed.), *Queering the Renaissance* (pp. 280–309). Durham, NC: Duke University Press.

Matchim, Y., Armer, J. M., & Stewart, B. R. (2008). A qualitative study of participants' perceptions of the effect of mindfulness meditation practice on self-care and overall well-being. *The Official Journal of the International Orem Society, 16*(2), 46–53.

Mayer, J. D., & Salovey, P. (1997). What is emotional intelligence? In P. Salovey & D. J. Sluyter (Eds), *Emotional Development and Emotional Intelligence* (pp. 3–31). New York: Basic Books.

Mayer, J. D., Salovey, P., & Caruso, D. R. (2008). Emotional intelligence: New ability or eclectic traits? *American Psychologist, 63*(6), 503–517.

McKinlay, A. (2010). Performativity and the politics of identity: Putting Butler to work. *Critical Perspectives on Accounting, 21*(3), 232–242.

McMahan, D. L. (2004). Modernity and the early discourse of scientific buddhism. *Journal of the American Academy of Religion, 72*(4), 897–933.

McManus, S., Meltzer, H., Brugha, T., Bebbington, P., & Jenkins, R. (2009). *Adult Psychiatric Morbidity in England, 2007: Results of a Household Survey.* London: NHS Information Centre for Health and Social Care.

Mejía, X. E. (2005). Gender matters: Working with adult male survivors of trauma. *Journal of Counseling & Development, 83*(1), 29–40.

Meltzer, H., Bebbington, P., Brugha, T., Jenkins, R., McManus, S., & Stansfeld, S. (2010). Job insecurity, socio-economic circumstances and depression. *Psychological Medicine, 40*(08), 1401–1407.

Merriam, S. B., & Heuer, B. (1996). Meaning-making, adult learning and development: A model with implications for practice. *International Journal of Lifelong Education, 15*(4), 243–255.

Messner, M. (1993). 'Changing men' and feminist politics in the United States. *Theory and Society, 22*(5), 723–737.

Meth, R. L., Pasick, R. S., Gordon, B., Allen, J. A., Feldman, L. B., & Gordon, S. (1991). *Men in Therapy: The Challenge of Change.* London: Guilford Press.

Mikulas, W. I. (1990). Mindfulness, self-control, and personal growth. In M. G. T. Kwee (Ed.), *Psychotherapy, Meditation, and Health* (pp. 151–164). London: East West Publications.

Mill, J. S. (1863). *Utilitarianism, Liberty and Representative Government.* London: Dent & Sons.

Mills, T. C., Paul, J., Stall, R., Pollack, L., Canchola, J., Chang, Y. J., et al. (2004). Distress and depression in men who have sex with men: The urban men's health study. *The American Journal of Psychiatry, 161*(2), 278–285.

Ministry of Justice (2012). Statistics on Women and the Criminal Justice System 2011.

The Mirror (2011). Meditate to Live Longer. 19 May 2011, retrieved 16 February 2013, from www.mirror.co.uk/lifestyle/sex-relationships/meditate-to-live-longer-129309

Mirsky, A., Anthony, B., Duncan, C., Ahearn, M., & Kellam, S. (1991). Analysis of the elements of attention: A neuropsychological approach. *Neuropsychology Review, 2*(2), 109–145.

Mischel, W. (1975). A social-learning view of sex differences in behavior. In E. E. Maccoby (Ed.), *The Development of Sex Differences* (pp. 56–81). Stanford, CA: Stanford University Press.

Money, J., Hampson, J. G., & Hampson, J. L. (1957). Imprinting and the establishment of gender role. *Archives of Neurology and Psychiatry, 77*(3), 333–336.

Moon, D. G., Hecht, M. L., Jackson, K. M., & Spellers, R. E. (1999). Ethnic and gender differences and similarities in adolescent drug use and refusals of drug offers. *Substance Use & Misuse, 34*(8), 1059–1083.

Moore, T. M., & Stuart, G. L. (2005). A review of the literature on masculinity and partner violence. *Psychology of Men & Masculinity, 6*(1), 46–61.

Morrongiello, B. A., & Dawber, T. (2000). Mothers' responses to sons and daughters engaging in injury-risk behaviors on a playground: Implications for sex differences in injury rates. *Journal of Experimental Child Psychology, 76*(2), 89–103.

Mosher, D. L., & Tomkins, S. S. (1988). Scripting the macho man: Hypermasculine socialization and enculturation. *Journal of Sex Research, 25*(1), 60–84.

Moss-Racusin, C. A., Phelan, J. E., & Rudman, L. A. (2010). When men break the gender rules: Status incongruity and backlash against modest men. *Psychology of Men & Masculinity, 11*(2), 140–151.

Müller, H. J., & Rabbitt, P. M. (1989). Reflexive and voluntary orienting of visual attention: Time course of activation and resistance to interruption. *Journal of Experimental Psychology: Human Perception and Performance, 15*(2), 315–330. doi: 10.1037/0096-1523.15.2.315

Munn, J. (2008). The hegemonic male and Kosovar nationalism, 2000–2005. *Men and Masculinities, 10*(4), 440–456.

Nagel, T. (1974). What is it like to be a bat? *The Philosophical Review, 83*(4), 435–450.

Nakhaie, R., & Arnold, R. (2010). A four year (1996–2000) analysis of social capital and health status of Canadians: The difference that love makes. *Social Science & Medicine, 71*(5), 1037–1044.

National Institute for Health and Clinical Excellence [NICE] (2004). Depression: Management of Depression in Primary and Secondary Care. *Clinical Guideline 23.*

Nayak, A. (2006). Displaced masculinities: Chavs, youth and class in the post-industrial city. *Sociology, 40*(5), 813–831.

Nayak, A., & Kehily, M. J. (2006). Gender undone: Subversion, regulation and embodiment in the work of Judith Butler. *British Journal of Sociology of Education, 27*(4), 459–472.

Neff, K. D. (2003). Self-compassion: An alternative conceptualization of a healthy attitude toward oneself. *Self and Identity, 2*(2), 85–101.

Neff, K. D., Kirkpatrick, K. L., & Rude, S. S. (2007). Self-compassion and adaptive psychological functioning. *Journal of Research in Personality, 41*(1), 139–154.

Neimeyer, R. A. (2006). Widowhood, grief and the quest for meaning. In D. S. Carr, R. M. Ness, & C. B. Wortman (Eds), *Spousal Bereavement in Late Life* (pp. 227–252). New York: Springer Publishing.

Neumann, I. D. (2008). Brain oxytocin: A key regulator of emotional and social behaviours in both females and males. *Journal of Neuroendocrinology, 20*(6), 858–865.

Neustadter, R. (2004). Archetypical life scripts in memoirs of childhood: Heaven, hell and purgatory. *Auto/Biography, 12*, 236–259.

The New Scientist (2011). Heal Thyself: Meditate. 30 August 2011, retrieved 16 February 2013, from www.newscientist.com/article/mg21128271.900-heal-thyself-meditate.html

Nhat-Tu, B. T. (2013). Human Existence in Terms of Six Elements (Cha-Dhaatu). Retrieved from www.truehappiness.ws/Human_Existence_in_Terms_of_Six Elements.html

NHS Information Centre (2011). In-Patients Formally Detained in Hospitals under the Mental Health Act, 1983 – and Patients Subject to Supervised Community Treatment, Annual figures, England, 2010/11.

Nietzsche, F. (1886). *Beyond Good and Evil* (M. Faber, Trans.). Oxford: Oxford World's Classics.

Nightingale, A. (2006). The nature of gender: Work, nature and environment. *Environment and Planning D: Society and Space, 24*(2), 165–185.

Nolen-Hoeksema, S. (1987). Sex differences in unipolar depression: Evidence and theory. *Psychological Bulletin, 101*(2), 259–282.

Nolen-Hoeksema, S. (1991). Responses to depression and their effects on the duration of depressive episodes. *Journal of Abnormal Psychology, 100*(4), 569–582.

Nolen-Hoeksema, S. (2001). Gender differences in depression. *Current Directions in Psychological Science, 10*(5), 173–176.

Noone, J. H., & Stephens, C. (2008). Men, masculine identities, and health care utilisation. *Sociology of Health and Illness, 30*(5), 711–725.

Obadia, L. (2008). The economies of health in Western Buddhism: A case study of a Tibetan Buddhist group in France. In D. C. Wood (Ed.), *The Economics of Health and Wellness: Anthropological Perspectives* (pp. 227–259). Oxford: JAI Press.

Obermeyer, C. M., Schulein, M., Hardon, A., Sievert, L. L., Price, K., Santiago, A. C., et al. (2004). Gender and medication use: An exploratory, multi-site study. *Women & Health, 39*(4), 57–73.

O'Connor, D. B., Archer, J., Hair, W. M., & Wu, F. C. W. (2001). Activational effects of testosterone on cognitive function in men. *Neuropsychologia, 39*(13), 1385–1394.

Office for National Statistics [ONS] (2011a). Atlas of Deprivation 2010.

Office for National Statistics (2011b). Civil Service Statistics 2011.

Office for National Statistics (2012a). Alcohol-Related Deaths in the UK, 2010.

Office for National Statistics (2012b). Measuring National Well-Being – Health.

Office for National Statistics (2012c). Statistical Bulletin: Deaths Related to Drug Poisoning in England and Wales, 2011.

Office for National Statistics (2012d). Suicide Rates in the United Kingdom, 2006 to 2010.

Office for National Statistics (2013). Statistical Bulletin: Suicides in the United Kingdom, 2011.

Oliffe, J. L., & Phillips, M. J. (2008). Men, depression and masculinities: A review and recommendations. *Journal of Men's Health, 5*(3), 194–202.

O'Neil, J. M., Good, G. E., & Holmes, S. (1995). Fifteen years of research on men's gender role conflict: New paradigms for empirical research. In R. F. Levant & W. S. Pollack (Eds), *A New Psychology of Men* (pp. 164–206). New York: Basic Books.

Ong, L. (2007). The kinesthetic Buddha, human form and function – Part 1: Breathing Torso. *Journal of Bodywork and Movement Therapies, 11*(3), 214–222.

O'Sullivan, S. (2001). Writing on art (case study: the Buddhist puja). *Parallax, 7*(4), 115–121.

Overholser, J. C. (1993). Elements of the Socratic method: Systematic questioning. *Psychotherapy: Theory, Research, Practice, Training, 30*(1), 67–74.

Oxford English Dictionary (1971). Oxford: Oxford University Press.

Paechter, C. (2003). Masculinities and femininities as communities of practice. *Women's Studies International Forum, 26*(1), 69–77.

Park, C. L. (2005). Religion as a meaning-making framework in coping with life stress. *Journal of Social Issues, 61*(4), 707–729.

Parker, A. (2006). Lifelong learning to labour: Apprenticeship, masculinity and communities of practice. *British Educational Research Journal, 32*(5), 687–701.

Patel, V. L., Arocha, J. F., & Kushniruk, A. W. (2002). Patients' and physicians' understanding of health and biomedical concepts: Relationship to the design of EMR systems. *Journal of Biomedical Informatics, 35*(1), 8–16.

Perez-De-Albeniz, A., & Holmes, J. (2000). Meditation: Concepts, effects and uses in therapy. *International Journal of Psychotherapy, 5*(1), 49–58.

Peterson, C., Park, N., & Seligman, M. P. (2005). Orientations to happiness and life satisfaction: The full life versus the empty life. *Journal of Happiness Studies, 6*(1), 25–41.

Petrides, K. V., & Furnham, A. (2003). Trait emotional intelligence: Behavioural validation in two studies of emotion recognition and reactivity to mood induction. *European Journal of Personality, 17*(1), 39–57.

Pittau, M. G., Zelli, R., & Gelman, A. (2010). Economic disparities and life satisfaction in European regions. *Social Indicators Research, 96*(2), 339–361.

Pleck, J. H. (1995). The gender role strain paradigm: An update. In R. F. Levant & W. S. Pollack (Eds), *A New Psychology of Men* (pp. 11–32). New York: Basic Books.

Plexico, L. W., Manning, W. H., & Levitt, H. (2009). Coping responses by adults who stutter: Part I. Protecting the self and others. *Journal of Fluency Disorders, 34*(2), 87–107.

Pollack, W. S. (1998). Mourning, melancholia, and masculinity: Recognizing and treating depression in men. In W. S. Pollack & R. F. Levant (Eds), *New Psychotherapy for Men* (pp. 147–166). Hoboken, NJ: John Wiley and Sons.

Pollack, W. S. (2006). The 'war' for boys: Hearing 'real boys" voices, healing their pain. *Professional Psychology: Research and Practice, 37*(2), 190–195.

Pollard, E. L., & Davidson, L. (2001). Foundations of Child Wellbeing. *Action Research in Family and Early Childhood*. Paris: UNESCO.

Popp-Baier, U. (2002). Conversion as a social construction: A narrative approach to conversion research. In C. A. M. Hermans, G. Immink, A. De Jong, & J. Van Der Lans (Eds), *Social Constructionism and Theology* (pp. 41–62). Netherlands: Koninklijke.

Posner, M. I., & Petersen, S. E. (1990). The attention system of the human brain. *Annual Review of Neuroscience, 13*(1), 25–42.

Pullen, A., & Simpson, R. (2009). Managing difference in feminized work: Men, otherness and social practice. *Human Relations, 62*(4), 561–587.

Rabinowitz, F. E., & Cochran, S. V. (2008). Men and therapy. *Clinical Case Studies, 7*(6), 575–591.

Rafal, R. D., & Posner, M. I. (1987). Deficits in human visual spatial attention following thalamic lesions. *Proceedings of the National Academy of Sciences, 84*(20), 7349–7353.

Raffone, A., & Srinivasan, N. (2010). The exploration of meditation in the neuroscience of attention and consciousness. *Cognitive Processing, 11*(1), 1–7.

Rail, G. (1998). Introduction. In G. Rail (Ed.), *Sport and Postmodern Times*. Albany: New York Press.

Ratner, C., & El-Badwi, E. S. (2011). A cultural psychological theory of mental illness, supported by research in Saudi Arabia. *Journal of Social Distress and the Homeless, 20*(3), 217–274.

Ravitz, P., Maunder, R., Hunter, J., Sthankiya, B., & Lancee, W. (2010). Adult attachment measures: A 25-year review. *Journal of Psychosomatic Research, 69*(4), 419–432.

Redden, G. (2005). The new age: Towards a market model. *Journal of Contemporary Religion, 20*(2), 231–246.

Reed, J., & Ones, D. S. (2006). The effect of acute aerobic exercise on positive activated affect: A meta-analysis. *Psychology of Sport and Exercise, 7*(5), 477–514.

Resnick, S., Warmoth, A., & Serlin, I. A. (2001). The humanistic psychology and positive psychology connection: Implications for psychotherapy. *Journal of Humanistic Psychology, 41*(1), 73–101.

Richins, M. L., & Dawson, S. (1992). A consumer values orientation for materialism and its measurement: Scale development and validation. *Journal of Consumer Research, 19*(3), 303–316.

Ricoeur, P. (1981). *Hermeneutics and the Human Sciences* (J. B. Thompson, Trans.). Cambridge: Cambridge University Press.

Ridge, D., Williams, I., Anderson, J., & Elford, J. (2008). Like a prayer: The role of spirituality and religion for people living with HIV in the UK. *Sociology of Health & Illness, 30*(3), 413–428.

Riesman, D., Glazer, N., & Denney, R. (1961). *The Lonely Crowd: A Study of the Changing American Character*. New Haven, CT: Yale University Press.

Ringrose, J. (2006). A new universal mean girl: Examining the discursive construction and social regulation of a new feminine pathology. *Feminism & Psychology, 16*(4), 405–424.

Roberts, J., & Clement, A. (2007). Materialism and satisfaction with over-all quality of life and eight life domains. *Social Indicators Research, 82*(1), 79–92.

Roberts, P. (1993). Social control and the censure(s) of sex. *Crime, Law and Social Change, 19*(2), 171–186.

Robertson, S., & Williamson, P. (2005). Men and health promotion in the UK: Ten years further on? *Health Education Journal, 64*(4), 293–301.

Roemer, L., & Borkovec, T. D. (1994). Effects of suppressing thoughts about emotional material. *Journal of Abnormal Psychology, 103*(3), 467–474.

Rogers, C. (1951). *Client-Centered Therapy: Its Current Practice, Implications and Theory*. London: Constable.

Rogers, C. R. (1961). *On Becoming a Person: A Therapist's View of Psychotherapy*. New York: Houghton Mifflin.

Ross, C. E. (2000). Neighborhood disadvantage and adult depression. *Journal of Health and Social Behavior, 41*(2), 177–187.

Ross-Smith, A., & Kornberger, M. (2004). Gendered rationality? A genealogical exploration of the philosophical and sociological conceptions of rationality, masculinity and organization. *Gender, Work & Organization, 11*(3), 280–305.

Russell, J. A., Weiss, A., & Mendelsohn, G. A. (1989). Affect grid: A single-item scale of pleasure and arousal. *Journal of Personality and Social Psychology, 57*(3), 493–502.

Ryan, R. M., & Deci, E. L. (2000). Self-determination theory and the facilitation of intrinsic motivation, social development, and well-being. *American Psychologist, 55*(1), 68–78.

Ryan, R. M., & Deci, E. L. (2001). On happiness and human potentials: A review of research on hedonic and eudaimonic well-being. *Annual Review of Psychology, 52*(1), 141–166.

Ryan, R. M., Huta, V., & Deci, E. (2008). Living well: A self-determination theory perspective on eudaimonia. *Journal of Happiness Studies, 9*(1), 139–170.

Ryan, T. (2001). *Prayer of Heart and Body: Meditation and Yoga as Christian Spiritual Practice*. Mahwah, NJ: Paulist Press.

Ryff, C. D., & Keyes, C. L. M. (1995). The structure of psychological well-being revisited. *Journal of Personality and Social Psychology, 69*(4), 719–727.

Ryff, C. D., & Singer, B. (1998). The contours of positive human health. *Psychological Inquiry, 9*(1), 1–28.

Saewyc, E. M., Skay, C. L., Hynds, P., Pettingell, S., Bearinger, L. H., Resnick, M. D., & Reis, E. (2008). Suicidal ideation and attempts in North American school-based surveys: Are bisexual youth at increasing risk? *Journal of LGBT Health Research, 3*(2), 25–36.

Said, E. W. (1995). *Orientalism: Western Conceptions of the Orient.* London: Penguin.

Salovey, P., & Mayer, J. D. (1989). Emotional intelligence. *Imagination, Cognition and Personality, 9*(3), 185–211.

Salzberg, S. (2004). *Loving-Kindness: The Revolutionary Art of Happiness.* Boston: Shambhala Publications.

Sandlund, E., & Norlander, T. (2000). The effects of Tai Chi Chuan relaxation and exercise on stress responses and well-being: An overview of research. *International Journal of Stress Management, 7*(2), 139–149.

Sangharakshita (1993). *Forty Three Years Ago: Reflections on My Bhikkhu Ordination.* London: Windhorse Publications.

Sangharakshita, U. (1997). *The Rainbow Road.* Glasgow: Windhorse Publications.

Sarrazin, J.-C., Cleeremans, A., & Haggard, P. (2008). How do we know what we are doing? Time, intention and awareness of action. *Consciousness and Cognition, 17*(3), 602–615.

Sartre, J. P. (1943). *Being and Nothingness.* New York: Gramercy Books.

Saso, M. (1990). *Tantric Art and Meditation.* Honolulu, Hawaii: University of Hawaii Press.

Savin-Baden, M., & Niekerk, L. V. (2007). Narrative inquiry: Theory and practice. *Journal of Geography in Higher Education, 31*(3), 459–472.

Sawni, A., & Breuner, C. C. (2012). Complementary, holistic, and integrative medicine: Depression, sleep disorders, and substance abuse. *Pediatrics in Review, 33*(9), 422–425.

Schak, D. C. (2008). Gender and Buddhism in Taiwan. *Hsuan Chuang Journal of Buddhist Studies, 9.*

Schalow, P. G. (1992). Kukai and the tradition of male love in Japanese Buddhism. In J. I. Cabezón (Ed.), *Buddhism, Sexuality and Gender* (pp. 215–230). Albany: State University of New York Press.

Scherer, B. (2011). Macho Buddhism: Gender and sexism in the Diamond way. *Religion and Gender, 1*(1), 85–103.

Schmid Mast, M., Sieverding, M., Esslen, M., Graber, K., & Jäncke, L. (2008). Masculinity causes speeding in young men. *Accident Analysis & Prevention, 40*(2), 840–842.

Schmidt-Wilk, J., Alexander, C., & Swanson, G. (1996). Developing consciousness in organizations: The transcendental meditation program in business. *Journal of Business and Psychology, 10*(4), 429–444.

Schonert-Reichl, K. A., & Lawlor, M. S. (2010). The effects of a mindfulness-based education program on pre- and early adolescents' well-being and social and emotional competence. *Mindfulness, 1,* 137–151.

Schwartz, J. P., & Waldo, M. (2003). Reducing gender role conflict among men attending partner abuse prevention groups. *The Journal for Specialists in Group Work, 28*(4), 355–369.

Scully, J. A., Tosi, H., & Banning, K. (2000). Life event checklists: Revisiting the social readjustment rating scale after 30 years. *Educational and Psychological Measurement, 60*(6), 864–876.

Seale, C., & Charteris-Black, J. (2008). The interaction of class and gender in illness narratives. *Sociology, 42*(3), 453–469.

Seligman, M. E. P. (2002). *Authentic Happiness*. New York: Free Press.

Seligman, M. E. P., & Csikszentmihalyi, M. (2000). Positive psychology: An introduction. *American Psychologist, 55*(1), 5–14.

Seligman, M. E. P., Steen, T. A., Park, N., & Peterson, C. (2005). Positive psychology progress: Empirical validation of interventions. *American Psychologist, 60*(5), 410–421.

Seligman, M. E. P., Rashid, T., & Parks, A. C. (2006). Positive psychotherapy. *American Psychologist, 61*(8), 774–788.

Shapiro, D. H. (1992). Adverse effects of meditation: A preliminary investigation of long-term meditators. *International Journal of Psychosomatics, 39*(1–4), 62–67.

Shapiro, D. H. (1994). Examining the content and context of meditation: A challenge for psychology in the areas of stress management, psychotherapy, and religion/values. *Journal of Humanistic Psychology, 34*(4), 101–135.

Shapiro, S. L., Carlson, L. E., Astin, J. A., & Freedman, B. (2006). Mechanisms of mindfulness. *Journal of Clinical Psychology, 62*(3), 373–386.

Shin, D. C., & Johnson, D. M. (1978). Avowed happiness as an overall assessment of the quality of life. *Social Indicators Research, 5*(1–4), 475–492.

Shiner, M., Scourfield, J., Fincham, B., & Langer, S. (2009). When things fall apart: Gender and suicide across the life-course. *Social Science & Medicine, 69*(5), 738–746.

Siderits, M. (2003). *Personal Identity and Buddhist Philosophy: Empty Persons.* Aldershot: Ashgate Publishing.

Siegel, D. J. (2007). *The Mindful Brain.* New York: Norton.

Siegrist, J. (1996). Adverse health effects of high-effort/low-reward conditions. *Journal of Occupational Health Psychology, 1*(1), 27–41.

Simon, P., Gonzalez, E., Ginsburg, D., Abrams, J., & Fielding, J. (2009). Physical activity promotion: A local and state health department perspective. *Preventive Medicine, 49*(4), 297–298.

Smith, J. A., Braunack-Mayer, A., Wittert, G., & Warin, M. (2007). 'I've been independent for so damn long!': Independence, masculinity and aging in a help seeking context. *Journal of Aging Studies, 21*(4), 325–335.

Smith, J. M., & Alloy, L. B. (2009). A roadmap to rumination: A review of the definition, assessment, and conceptualization of this multifaceted construct. *Clinical Psychology Review, 29*(2), 116–128.

Smith, S. E. (2008). *Buddhism, diversity and 'race': Multiculturalism and Western convert Buddhist movements in East London – a qualitative study.* (PhD), Goldsmiths, University of London, Goldsmiths Research Online. Retrieved from http://eprints.gold.ac.uk/2553

Smith, T. E., & Leaper, C. (2006). Self-perceived gender typicality and the peer context during adolescence. *Journal of Research on Adolescence, 16*(1), 91–104.

Smokowski, P. R. (1998). Prevention and intervention strategies for promoting resilience in disadvantaged children. *Social Service Review, 72*(3), 337–364.

Soroka, S. N., Helliwell, J. F., & Johnston, R. (2003). Measuring and modelling trust. In F. Kay & R. Johnston (Eds), *Diversity, Social Capital and the Welfare State.* Vancouver, BC: University of British Columbia Press.

Spaaij, R. (2008). Men like us, boys like them: Violence, masculinity, and collective identity in football hooliganism. *Journal of Sport & Social Issues, 32*(4), 369–392.

Spira, A. P., Zvolensky, M. J., Eifert, G. H., & Feldner, M. T. (2004). Avoidance-oriented coping as a predictor of panic-related distress: A test using biological challenge. *Journal of Anxiety Disorders, 18*(3), 309–323.

Stanton, A. L., Kirk, S. B., Cameron, C. L., & Danoff-Burg, S. (2000). Coping through emotional approach: Scale construction and validation. *Journal of Personality and Social Psychology, 78*(6), 1150–1169.

Stobbe, L. (2005). Doing machismo: Legitimating speech acts as a selection discourse. *Gender, Work & Organization, 12*(2), 105–123.

Strauss, A., & Corbin, J. (1998). *Basics of Qualitative Research: Techniques and Procedures for Developing Grounded Theory* (2nd ed.). Thousand Oaks, CA: Sage.

Strunk, D. R., & Adler, A. D. (2009). Cognitive biases in three prediction tasks: A test of the cognitive model of depression. *Behaviour Research and Therapy, 47*(1), 34–40.

Stutzer, A., & Frey, B. S. (2006). Does marriage make people happy, or do happy people get married? *The Journal of Socio-Economics, 35*(2), 326–347.

Subhuti, D. (1994). *Sangharakshita: A New Voice in the Buddhist Tradition*. Glasgow: Windhorse Publications.

Suh, E., Diener, E., & Fujita, F. (1996). Events and subjective well-being: Only recent events matter. *Journal of Personality and Social Psychology, 70*(5), 1091–1102.

Tagg, B. (2008). 'Imagine, a man playing netball!': Masculinities and sport in New Zealand. *International Review for the Sociology of Sport, 43*(4), 409–430.

Teasdale, J. D. (1988). Cognitive vulnerability to persistent depression. *Cognition & Emotion, 2*(3), 247–274.

Teasdale, J. D., Segal, Z. V., Williams, J. M. G., Ridgeway, V. A., Soulsby, J. M., & Lau, M. A. (2000). Prevention of relapse/recurrence in major depression by mindfulness-based cognitive therapy. *Journal of Consulting and Clinical Psychology, 68*(4), 615–623.

Teasdale, J. D., Segal, S. V., & Williams, J. M. G. (2003). Mindfulness training and problem formulation. *Clinical Psychology: Science and Practice, 10*(2), 157–160.

Tedeschi, R. G., & Calhoun, L. G. (2004). Posttraumatic growth: Conceptual foundations and empirical evidence. *Psychological Inquiry, 15*(1), 1–18.

Teixeira, M. E. (2008). Meditation as an intervention for chronic pain: An integrative review. *Holistic Nursing Practice, 22*(4), 225–234.

Tennant, C. (2002). Life events, stress and depression: A review of recent findings. *Australian and New Zealand Journal of Psychiatry, 36*(2), 173–182.

Thomas, E. J. (2000). *The Life of Buddha as Legend and History*. New York: Dover.

Thompson, R. A. (1994). Emotional regulation: A theme in search of a definition. *Monographs of the Society for Research in Child Development, 59*(2–3), 25–52.

Thrangu, K. (1993). *The Practice of Tranquility and Insight: A Guide to Tibetan Buddhist Meditation* (R. Roberts, Trans.). Boston: Shambhala Publications.

Thurnell-Read, T., & Parker, A. (2008). Men, masculinities and firefighting: Occupational identity, shop-floor culture and organisational change. *Emotion, Space and Society, 1*(2), 127–134.

Tillich, P. (1952). *The Courage to Be*. Glasgow: William Collins.

Tischler, L., Biberman, J., & McKeage, R. (2002). Linking emotional intelligence, spirituality and workplace performance: Definitions, models and ideas for research. *Journal of Managerial Psychology, 17*(3), 203–218.

Tolle, E. (2004). *The Power of Now: A Guide to Spiritual Enlightenment.* USA: New World Library.

Travis, F., & Shear, J. (2010). Focused attention, open monitoring and automatic self-transcending: Categories to organize meditations from Vedic, Buddhist and Chinese traditions. *Consciousness and Cognition, 19*(4), 1110–1118.

Turner, R. J., & Lloyd, D. A. (2004). Stress burden and the lifetime incidence of psychiatric disorder in young adults: Racial and ethnic contrasts. *Archives of General Psychiatry, 61*(5), 481–488.

Tyner, J. A. (2008). *The Killing of Cambodia: Geography, Genocide, and the Unmaking of Space.* Aldershot: Ashgate Publishing.

Uecker, J. E., Regnerus, M. D., & Vaaler, M. L. (2007). Losing my religion: The social sources of religious decline in early adulthood. *Social Forces, 85*(4), 1667–1692.

Universities UK (2012). UUK Members: List of University Heads. Retrieved 27 December 2012, from www.universitiesuk.ac.uk/AboutUs/WhoWeAre/Pages/Members.aspx

Underwood, L. (1999). Daily spiritual experiences. In *Multidimensional Measurement of Religiousness/Spirituality for Use in Health Research: A Report of the Fetzer Institute/National Institute on Aging Working Group* (pp. 11–18). Washington, DC: National Institute on Aging.

United Nations Educational, Social and Cultural Organization [UNESCO] (1997). Lumbini: UNESCO World Heritage Site. Retrieved 16 February 2013, from www.unesco.org/new/index.php?id=69625.

Uppal, S. (2006). Impact of the timing, type and severity of disability on the subjective well-being of individuals with disabilities. *Social Science & Medicine, 63*(2), 525–539.

Vajragupta (2010). *The Triratna Story: Behind the Scenes of a New Buddhist Movement.* Cambridge: Windhorse Publications.

Van Nortwick, T. (2008). *Imagining Men: Ideals of Masculinity in Ancient Greek Culture.* Westport, CT: Praeger Publishers.

Varenne, J. (1977). *Yoga and the Hindu Tradition.* Chicago: University of Chicago Press.

Veal, A. J. (1993). The concept of lifestyle: A review. *Leisure Studies, 12*(4), 233–252.

Vessantara (2002). *Meeting the Buddhas: A Guide to Buddhas, Bohisattvas, and Tantric Deities.* Birmingham: Windhorse Publications.

Vettese, L. C., Toneatto, T., Stea, J. N., Nguyen, L., & Wang, J. J. (2009). Do mindfulness meditation participants do their homework? And does it make a difference? A review of the empirical evidence. *Journal of Cognitive Psychotherapy, 23*(3), 198–225.

Vincent, K. S. (1988). The longing for total revolution: Philosophic sources of social discontent from Rousseau to Marx and Nietzsche. *History of European Ideas, 9*(3), 364–365.

Vinnicombe, S., Sealy, R., Graham, J., & Doldor, E. (2010). The Female FTSE 100 Board Report: Opening up the Process. Cranfield University School of Management.

Vishvapani, D. (2001). Perceptions of the FWBO in British Buddhism. *Western Buddhist Review, 3.*

Walsh, R., & Shapiro, S. L. (2006). The meeting of meditative disciplines and western psychology: A mutually enriching dialogue. *American Psychologist, 61*(3), 227–239.

Warner, J., McKeown, E., Griffin, M., Johnson, K., Ramsay, A., Cort, C., & King, M. (2004). Rates and predictors of mental illness in gay men, lesbians and bisexual men and women: Results from a survey based in England and Wales. *British Journal of Psychiatry, 185*(6), 479–485.

Webb, E., Ashton, C. H., Kelly, P., & Kamali, F. (1996). Alcohol and drug use in UK university students. *The Lancet, 348*(9032), 922–925.

Wegner, D. M., & Gold, D. B. (1995). Fanning old flames: Emotional and cognitive effects of suppressing thoughts of a past relationship. *Journal of Personality and Social Psychology, 68*(5), 782–792.

Weich, S., Nazroo, J., Sproston, K., McManus, S., Blanchard, M., Erens, B., et al. (2004). Common mental disorders and ethnicity in England: The EMPIRIC study. *Psychological Medicine, 34*(8), 1543–1551.

West, C., & Zimmerman, D. H. (1987). Doing gender. *Gender & Society, 1*(2), 125–151.

Wetherell, M., & Edley, N. (1999). Negotiating hegemonic masculinity: Imaginary positions and psycho-discursive practices. *Feminism & Psychology, 9*(3), 335–356.

White, H. (1987). *The Content of the Form: Narrative Discourse and Historical Representation*. Baltimore: Johns Hopkins University Press.

Wilber, K. (1995). *Sex, Ecology, Spirituality: The Spirit of Evolution*. Boston: Shambhala Publications.

Wildegren, G. (1961). Researches in Syrian mysticism: Mystical experiences and Spiritual exercises. *Numen: International Review for the History of Religions, 8*, 161–198.

Wilhelm, D., & Koopman, P. (2006). The makings of maleness: Towards an integrated view of male sexual development. *Nature Reviews Genetics, 7*(8), 620.

Winkler, D., Pjrek, E., & Kasper, S. (2006). Gender-specific symptoms of depression and anger attacks. *The Journal of Men's Health & Gender, 3*(1), 19–24.

Witt, S. D. (2000). The influence of television on children's gender role socialization. *Childhood Education, 76*(5), 322–324.

Wong, P. T., & Fry, P. S. (1998). *The Human Quest for Meaning*. Mahwah, NJ: Erlbaum.

Wood, A. M., Joseph, S., & Maltby, J. (2008). Gratitude uniquely predicts satisfaction with life: Incremental validity above the domains and facets of the five factor model. *Personality and Individual Differences, 45*(1), 49–54.

Woodruff, P. (2001). *Reverence: Renewing a Forgotten Virtue*. New York: Oxford University Press.

World Health Organization [WHO] (1948). Preamble to the Constitution of the World Health Organization as Adopted by the International Health Conference, New York, 19–22 June 1946; Signed on 22 July 1946 by the Representatives of 61 States (Official Records of the World Health Organization, no. 2, p. 100) and Entered into Force on 7 April 1948. World Health Organization.

World Health Organization (2012). What do we mean by 'sex' and 'gender'? *Gender, Women and Health*. Retrieved 28 December 2012, from www.who.int/gender/whatisgender/en/

Wortman, C. B., & Silver, R. C. (1989). The myths of coping with loss. *Journal of Consulting and Clinical Psychology, 57*(3), 349–357.

Wren, A. A., Wright, M. A., Carson, J. W., & Keefe, F. J. (2011). Yoga for persistent pain: New findings and directions for an ancient practice. *Pain, 152*(3), 477–480.

www.parliament.co.uk (2012). Her Majesty's Government. 17 December 2012, retrieved 27 December 2012, from www.parliament.uk/mps-lords-and-offices/government-and-opposition1/her-majestys-government/

Xu, S., & Connelly, F. M. (2009). Narrative inquiry for teacher education and development: Focus on English as a foreign language in China. *Teaching and Teacher Education, 25*(2), 219–227.

Yalom, I. (1980). *Existential Therapy*. New York: Basic Books.

Yorston, G. A. (2001). Mania precipitated by meditation: A case report and literature review. *Mental Health, Religion and Culture, 4*(2), 209–213.

Zahourek, R. P. (1998). Intentionality in transpersonal healing: Research and caregiver perspectives. *Complementary Health Practice Review, 4*(1), 11–27.

Zimbardo, P. G., & Boyd, J. N. (1999). Putting time in perspective: A valid, reliable individual-differences metric. *Journal of Personality and Social Psychology, 77*(6), 1271–1288.

Zylowska, L., Ackerman, D. L., Yang, M. H., Futrell, J. L., Horton, N. L., Hale, T. S., et al. (2008). Mindfulness meditation training in adults and adolescents with ADHD: A feasibility study. *Journal of Attention Disorders, 11*(6), 737–746.

Index

absorption, 31, 34, 71, 118, 139
abstinence, 23, 120, 148–50, 169, 172–3, 175
abuse, 14, 18, 41, 42, 44, 73
adam, 108–9, 113, 116, 126, 133, 134, 146, 149–50
adolescence, 6, 9, 42–9, 58, 72, 75, 113, 152, 158
adulthood, 6, 40, 41–3, 45–63, 51, 62, 72, 75, 153–4
affluence, 42, 47, 48, 69, 70, 77, 82, 173
agency, 20, 49–51, 53, 106, 134
  see also hyperagency
aggression, 1–3, 11, 13, 18, 42, 44, 47–50, 53, 60, 70, 79, 86, 107, 126, 127, 139, 155, 173
acceptance, 13, 30, 46, 49, 54–9, 62 111, 112, 117, 119, 125, 137–8, 167
achievement, *see* success
Addis, M., 57, 61, 62, 85, 87, 113, 122, 124, 127, 155, 156
affect, 26, 27, 57, 123, 129, 155
  see also emotions
aging, 60, 78, 111, 117
'Alan', 131
'Ali', 46, 60, 70, 86, 87, 92, 139, 147
alcohol
  abstinence/reduced consumption, 23, 120, 148–50, 169, 172–3, 175
  alcoholism/binge drinking, 2, 4, 42, 60, 149, 150, 155, 156
  as coping strategy, 8, 26, 27, 37–8, 67–8, 84–6, 124, 155
  death from, 60, 150
  as externalising behaviour, 60, 86, 155, 156
  gender differences, 2, 4, 60, 66, 87, 150

as masculine norm, 9, 37–8, 44, 53, 66, 70, 78, 80, 98, 149, 172–3
  pubs, 70, 78, 83, 84, 98, 150
  as remedy, 65, 67–8, 74, 85, 91
alexithymia, 57, 61, 105, 121, 152
altruism, 31
'Alvin', 42, 47, 48, 65, 69, 70, 78, 79, 104, 126, 147
American Psychiatric Association (APA), 24
anomalous experience, 28, 82, 108, 109, 116, 131–3, 140, 169
'Andrew', 51, 65, 100, 106, 118, 141, 146, 150
anger, 9, 59–63, 85, 86, 89, 106, 113, 130, 141, 143, 155, 156
anti-social behaviour, 11, 42, 79, 86, 126, 127, 139, 173
anxiety, 1, 24, 26, 35, 45, 56, 67, 79, 88, 90, 98, 106, 108, 133, 144, 148, 167, 169, 170
  see also mental health
arrest, 1, 79, 86
Asia, 79, 82, 83, 94–8, 108–10
at-risk youth, 42, 47, 48, 173–4
atheism, 73, 83, 85, 114
attachment, *see* upbringing
attention
  attitude of, 99, 110–16, 119, 125, 129, 145, 159, 162–5, 167
  behaviours of mind, *see* types of attention
  control, 143–6
  development of, 7, 92, 99–120, 123, 136, 150, 158–62, 167
  focussed attention (FA), 31, 71, 101, 103, 105, 111, 119, 159, 160, 167, 168
  form of, 99, 116–19, 133
  object of, 99, 104–10, 119, 159

attention – *continued*
  open monitoring (OM), 101, 102,
    104, 105, 119, 159, 160
  regulation of, 100, 143–6
  types of, 99–104, 119, 159
attitude
  acceptance, 13, 30, 46, 49, 111, 112,
    117, 119, 125, 137–8, 167
  compassion, 31, 109, 111–14, 118,
    128–31, 135, 140–41, 162–5,
    167, 170, 173
  devotion, 110, 111, 114–16,
    119, 159
  metta, 112–14, 119, 129–30, 132,
    140–41, 162–5
authenticity/inauthenticity, 29, 30,
    48, 49, 53–5, 58, 59, 78
autonomy, *see* independence
avoidance 13, 25–7, 51, 68, 155
awareness, *see* mindfulness

belief, 72, 73, 80, 81, 83, 85, 107–9,
    111, 114, 138–40, 166, 172
'Bill', 104
biology, 2, 3, 11–12, 38, 43, 83, 152
body, 41, 94, 99, 104, 105, 111, 116,
    117, 124, 133, 144, 146
boys, *see* childhood
bravado, 44, 45, 48, 49
breakdown, 7, 26, 43, 47, 56, 68, 74,
    84–91, 157
breath, 96, 101, 103, 104, 105, 117,
    160, 163, 165, 170
brother, 41, 48
Buddhism
  appeal of, 72, 73, 98, 111
  beliefs/discourses, 79, 107–9, 111,
    120, 138–40, 149, 166
  the Buddha, 82, 94–5, 97, 99, 109,
    110, 114–16
  community, 33, 35, 51, 52, 75, 84,
    98, 149–50, 169, 173, 175
  culture/society, 79, 95, 96
  the Dalai Lama, 96, 98, 109
  deities, 109, 110, 114
  dharma, 95, 114, 115
  the East, 74, 82
  enlightenment, 94–5, 97, 133
  Four noble truths, 95, 111

Friends of the Western Buddhism
    Order (FWBO), 96–8, 107,
    109, 112
  history of, 94–8
  Mahayana, 95, 96
  mandalas, 110
  'middle way,' 94, 114, 115
  mitras, 97
  monastery, *see* temple
  ordination, 96, 97, 107
  Pali, 96, 101, 112
  precepts, 120, 149
  pujas, *see* rituals
  as religion, 76
  rituals, 96, 110, 115
  sangha, *see* community
  Sangharakshita, 96
  Sanskrit, 94, 114, 115
  secularised, 97, 98, 176
  shrines, 110, 115–16, 159
  society/culture, 79, 95, 96
  as source of meaning, 72, 76, 82–4,
    109, 115–16, 126, 131–2, 149
  temple, 79, 82, 131
  theory of identity, 107–9, 138–40
  Therevada, 95, 96, 102
  'two arrows', 137–8
  in the West, 92, 93, 95–8
  Zen, 95, 96
bullying, *see* abuse
burnout, 69
Butler, J., 17–8, 20

calmness, 64, 71, 79, 87, 102, 123,
    125, 126, 132, 147
capital
  cultural, 48, 173
  economic, 173–4
  social, 32–4, 48, 120
capitalism, 54, 69–70, 172
careers, 35, 46, 47, 68, 69, 71–2, 77,
    80, 173
caring, 46, 69, 79, 86, 107, 112–14,
    130, 135, 154, 162–5, 167, 174
censure, 13, 18, 21, 41, 44, 46, 48, 49,
    54, 56, 78, 154, 172–3, 175
childhood, 4–6, 9, 38, 39–43, 58, 72,
    75, 81, 89, 113, 152, 158
choice, 68, 82–3, 143, 148–50

220   *Index*

Printed and bound by CPI Group (UK) Ltd, Croydon, CR0 4YY